ATRIAL FIBRILLATION AFTER CARDIAC SURGERY

Developments in Cardiovascular Medicine

198. Antoine Lafont, Eric Topol (eds.): *Arterial Remodeling: A Critical Factor in Restenosis.* 1997 ISBN 0-7923-8008-8
199. Michele Mercuri, David D. McPherson, Hisham Bassiouny, Seymour Glagov (eds.):*Non-Invasive Imaging of Atherosclerosis* ISBN 0-7923-8036-3
200. Walmor C. DeMello, Michiel J. Janse(eds.): *Heart Cell Communication in Health and Disease* ISBN 0-7923-8052-5
201. P.E. Vardas (ed.): *Cardiac Arrhythmias Pacing and Electrophysiology.* The Expert View. 1998 ISBN 0-7923-4908-3
202. E.E. van der Wall, P.K. Blanksma, M.G. Niemeyer, W. Vaalburg and H.J.G.M. Crijns (eds.) *Advanced Imaging in Coronary Artery Disease, PET, SPECT, MRI, IVUS, EBCT. 1998* ISBN 0-7923-5083-9
203. R.L. Wilensky (ed.) *Unstable Coronary Artery Syndromes, Pathophysiology, Diagnosis and Treatment. 1998.* ISBN 0-7923-8201-3
204. J.H.C. Reiber, E.E. van der Wall (eds.): *What's New in Cardiovascular Imaging?* 1998 ISBN 0-7923-5121-5
205. Juan Carlos Kaski, David W. Holt (eds.): *Myocardial Damage Early Detection by Novel Biochemical Markers. 1998.* ISBN 0-7923-5140-1
207. Gary F. Baxter, Derek M. Yellon, *Delayed Preconditioning and Adaptive Cardioprotection. 1998.* ISBN 0-7923-5259-9
208. Bernard Swynghedauw, *Molecular Cardiology for the Cardiologist, Second Edition* 1998. ISBN 0-7923-8323-0
209. Geoffrey Burnstock, James G.Dobson, Jr., Bruce T. Liang, Joel Linden (eds): *Cardiovascular Biology of Purines. 1998.* ISBN: 0-7923-8334-6
210. Brian D. Hoit, Richard A. Walsh (eds): *Cardiovascular Physiology in the Genetically Engineered Mouse.* 1998. ISBN: 0-7923-8356-7
211. Peter Whittaker, George S. Abela (eds.): *Direct Myocardial Revascularization: History, Methodology, Technology* 1998. ISBN: 0-7923-8398-2
212. C.A. Nienaber, R. Fattori (eds.): Diagnosis and Treatment of Aortic Diseases. 1999. ISBN: 0-7923-5517-2
213. Juan Carlos Kaski (ed.): *Chest Pain with Normal Coronary Angiograms: Pathogenesis, Diagnosis and Management.* 1999. ISBN: 0-7923-8421-0
214. P.A. Doevendans, R.S. Reneman and M. Van Bilsen (eds): *Cardiovascular Specific Gene Expression.* 1999 ISBN:0-7923-5633-0
215. G. Pons-Lladó, F. Carreras, X. Borrás, Subirana and L.J. Jiménez-Borreguero (eds.): *Atlas of Practical Cardiac Applications of MRI.* 1999 ISBN: 0-7923-5636-5
216. L.W. Klein, J.E. Calvin, *Resource Utilization in Cardiac Disease.* 1999. ISBN:0-7923-8509-8
217. R. Gorlin, G. Dangas, P. K. Toutouzas, M.M Konstadoulakis, *Contemporary Concepts in Cardiology, Pathophysiology and Clinical Management.*1999 ISBN:0-7923-8514-4
218. S. Gupta, J. Camm (eds.): *Chronic Infection, Chlamydia and Coronary Heart Disease.* 1999. ISBN:0-7923-5797-3
219. M. Rajskina: *Ventricular Fibrillation in Sudden Coronary Death.* 1999. ISBN:0-7923-8570-5
220. Z. Abedin, R. Conner: *Interpretation of Cardiac Arrhythmias: Self Assessment Approach.* 1999. ISBN:0-7923-8576-4
221. J. E. Lock, J.F. Keane, S. B. Perry: *Diagnostic and Interventional Catheterization In Congenital Heart Disease.* 2000. ISBN: 0-7923-8597-7

Previous volumes are still available

KLUWER ACADEMIC PUBLISHERS - DORDRECHT/BOSTON/LONDON

ATRIAL FIBRILLATION AFTER CARDIAC SURGERY

edited by

Jonathan S. Steinberg, MD

St. Luke's-Roosevelt Hospital Center
and
Columbia University College of Physicians and Surgeons

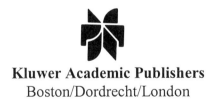

Kluwer Academic Publishers
Boston/Dordrecht/London

Distributors for North, Central and South America:
Kluwer Academic Publishers
101 Philip Drive
Assinippi Park
Norwell, Massachusetts 02061 USA

Distributors for all other countries:
Kluwer Academic Publishers Group
Distribution Centre
Post Office Box 322
3300 AH Dordrecht, THE NETHERLANDS

Library of Congress Cataloging-in-Publication Data

Atrial fibrillation after cardiac surgery/edited by Jonathan S. Steinberg.
    P. ; cm -- (Developments in cardiovascular medicine ; 222)
Includes index.
ISBN 0-7923-8655-8 (alk. Paper)
    1. Atrial fibrillation. 2. Heart--Surgery--Complications. I. Steinberg, Jonathan S.
II. Developments in cardiovascular medicine; v. 222
    [DNLM: 1. Atrial Fibrillation--complications. 2. Cardiac Surgical Procedures.
WG 330 A88165 1999]
RC685.A72 A8875 1999
617.4'1201--dc21   99-047095

Printed on acid-free paper.

Printed in the United States of America

Dedication

To my wife, Alice,
and my children, Rachel and Josh,
for their support and encouragement

Acknowledgement

The editor and authors would like to express their gratitude to
Janice Q. Pelegano
for her excellence in the process of editing and manuscript
preparation.

TABLE OF CONTENTS

Preface

Atrial fibrillation (AF) is the most common arrhythmic complication after cardiac surgery, and as in other settings, represents a serious therapeutic challenge. Its importance lies not only in the clinical complications that may ensue, or the patient discomfort frequently present, but also in its substantial impact on utilization of health care resources. This in large part arises from the product of the prevalence of AF and the additional length of stay necessary for its control and treatment; in today's environment, these issues have assumed near-paramount importance.

It is timely to review the specific subset of AF in the setting of cardiac surgery, and it remains useful to segregate this particular form of AF from AF in other clinical milieu. When AF occurs after cardiac surgery, there is an unusually narrow time window of risk; this unique situation lends itself to clinical intervention (risk stratification, prophylactic therapy and intensive surveillance) and clinical trial (large at-risk populations, high incidence, no loss of follow-up and well defined endpoint). However, AF after cardiac surgery has remained a persistent and stubborn problem that continues to attract the attention of individual practitioners and clinical investigators.

In this book, our authors will begin by describing the electrophysiologic abnormalities that are used to create AF (and other atrial arrhythmias) in the experimental animal model; these efforts have intriguing similarity to some of the changes that the atria undergo in routine cardiac surgery. The text will go on to describe several clinical observations that suggest the development of AF in the cardiac surgical patient has some similarities to AF in other clinical settings, but that there are also some unique features that indicate AF is at least partially mediated by special postoperative circumstances. When a patient leaves the operating room, the reader will learn of the fairly well circumscribed period of risk and a varied pattern of frequency, duration and consequences of AF. Next, one will read of the many studies that have examined which of the many cardiac surgical patients is at greatest risk based on clinical characteristics and also some new noninvasive tools. Of course, AF is not benign in its effect on hospital resources; it may eat up length of stay when the burden on physicians and staff is to move the patients out of the ICU, telemetry unit and hospital at faster and faster rates. This important subject will be discussed in detail.

How does one lessen the impact of AF? Two broad strategies will be discussed in detail. Several chapters deal with the results of different drug prophylactic schemes and with recent studies that have used atrial pacing to prevent AF. However, frequently one has to manage AF that has broken through despite attempts to prevent it and the options of cardioversion and anticoagulation will be addressed in detail.

Finally, AF also occurs after noncardiac surgery. Observations gathered in this group of patients may have particular relevance to the emerging use of minimally invasive cardiac surgery.

Cardiac surgery is performed on >500,000 patients each year in the U.S. alone. Because of its incidence, tenacity in the face of therapy, and consumption of precious health care resources, the focus on AF after cardiac surgery will persist among cardiologists, cardiac surgeons, anesthesiologists, nurses, hospital administrators and insurers. My colleagues and I have attempted to bring our readership a single source of information on this important problem. We hope to help health care professionals treat their patients optimally and to encourage researchers to continue their productive efforts.

1 EXPERIMENTAL ANIMAL MODELS OF ATRIAL ARRHYTHMIAS AND THEIR RELEVANCE TO POST-OPERATIVE ATRIAL ARRHYTHMIAS THAT OCCUR IN HUMANS UNERGOING CARDIAC SURGERY

Gregory K. Feld, MD,
University of California, San Diego, CA

1. Introduction

Atrial arrhythmias, such as atrial fibrillation (AFIB), atrial flutter (AFL) and atrial tachycardia (AT) are relatively common following cardiac surgery [1-2]. Patients undergoing cardiac surgery may be particularly prone to develop atrial arrhythmias for a variety of reasons, including the type of surgery performed, the presence of underlying heart disease and other associated medical conditions such as hypertension, hemodynamic instability or congestive heart failure, pulmonary insufficiency, associated pericardial inflammation, and the increased sympathetic and vagal nervous system activity that accompanies such surgery [1-2]. Post-operative atrial arrhythmias may cause significant symptoms including palpitations, shortness of breath, chest pain and even syncope due to the hemodynamic instability that often exists in this setting. If associated with a rapid ventricular response, post-operative atrial arrhythmias may cause ischemia or congestive heart failure, and in the case of atrial fibrillation thromboembolic stroke may even occur. The treatment, and perhaps more importantly the prevention of atrial arrhythmias following cardiac surgery is therefore critical. Fortunately, through extensive experimental and clinical studies significant progress has been made towards delineating the mechanisms and possible treatments for most atrial arrhythmias, including those that occur in the post-operative period following cardiac surgery.

For example, clinical studies in man have demonstrated that reentry is the electrophysiologic mechanism underlying many atrial arrhythmias, including AFIB, AFL and most forms of AT. In AFIB multiple reentrant circuits propagate throughout both the left and right atria [3-4], whereas in AFL a single reentrant circuit is confined to the right atrium [5-6], and in AT reentry circuits may develop around surgical incisions or prosthetic patch materials [7-8]. The delineation of these electrophysiologic mechanisms has been made possible in part by the use of percutaneous, catheter-based, multi-electrode mapping techniques [9-14], and in part by the use of intra-operative multi-electrode mapping techniques [15-16]. However, due to the invasive nature of the techniques required to study arrhythmias in man, animal models have also been created to better understand arrhythmia mechanism(s) and to develop safer and more effective treatments. These animal models, including several anatomical and functional reentry models of AFL and AT [17-25] and the pacing-induced models of AFIB [26-29], have electrophysiologic characteristics that are similar to human atrial arrhythmias, including those that occur following open-heart surgery for acquired or congenital heart disease.

This chapter will briefly review the relevant electrophysiologic characteristics of AFIB, AFL and AT, atrial arrhythmias that commonly occur in humans following cardiac surgery, and then describe in detail the experimental arrhythmia models that have been developed to study these clinically occurring arrhythmias.

2. Electrophysiologic Characteristics of Cardiac Arrhythmias That Commonly Occur Following Cardiac Surgery in Humans

Type 1AFL is a rapid, regular atrial tachycardia characterized by an inverted, saw-tooth flutter (F) wave pattern on surface electrocardiogram (ECG), at a rate ranging from 240-350 beats per minute. Type 1 AFL is due to a large reentry circuit in the right atrium that may rotate either in a counterclockwise (common form) or clockwise (uncommon form) direction [11-12]. The reentry circuit in type 1 AFL had been shown to have a fully excitable gap, during which both overt and concealed entrainment can be demonstrated [30-31]. Type 1 AFL can also be terminated by rapid overdrive atrial pacing [6]. Furthermore, there is a critical zone in the reentrant circuit where atrial flutter can be interrupted and cured by radiofrequency catheter ablation [32-33]. This critical zone is comprised of an isthmus of tissue between the inferior vena cava and tricuspid valve annulus (i.e. the TV-IVC isthmus), which has been shown to be more slowly conducting than other atrial tissue in the reentry circuit [34-35]. The TV-IVC isthmus has also been shown to be prone to development of unidirectional block, leading to initiation of reentry during induction of AFL by rapid atrial pacing [36-37]. Pharmacological termination of AFL in humans has been shown to be due to conduction block in the TV-IVC isthmus, which may occur either abruptly without cycle length oscillation, or following premature eccentric activation due to failure of lateral boundaries or reflected reentry in the reentry circuit [38]. During AFL double-potential electrograms have been recorded along the Eustachian ridge and the crista terminalis, suggesting that these anatomical structures form lines of block defining the posterior boundaries of the reentry circuit, while the tricuspid annulus forms the anterior boundary [39-44]. Thus, type 1 AFL is due to reentry around anatomically determined obstacles in the right atrium.

Type 2 AFL is characterized by an atypical F wave pattern on ECG, with atrial rates greater than 350 beats per minutes [45-46]. Type 2 AFL appears to be due to reentry around functionally determined lines of block. Such reentry circuits typically have only a partially excitable gap and may not be stable, thus accounting for the variability in F wave morphology of type 2 AFL between patients, or even between episodes in the same patient. As originally described by Waldo, et.al. in post-operative cardiac surgery patients, type 2 atrial flutter cannot be terminated by rapid overdrive atrial pacing [45]. Furthermore, since the arrhythmia circuit is functionally determined, localized catheter ablation is not an effective treatment for type 2 AFL.

Atrial tachycardias are rapid regular arrhythmias, characterized by discrete P waves with a distinct diastolic interval on ECG, at rates up to 240 beats per minute. Atrial tachycardias are due to reentry in many cases. In the post-operative cardiac surgery patient reentry may occur around a surgically created anatomical obstacle including an atriotomy scar or synthetic patch material [7-8]. Atrial tachycardia in the post-operative cardiac surgery patient, commonly called "scar tachycardia", usually involves a large reentry circuit with a fully excitable gap. Classical criteria for entrainment can usually be demonstrated during such AT. Double-potential electrograms may be recorded along an atriotomy scar identifying it as an anatomical obstacle. Typically, there will be a narrow isthmus of tissue between a scar or patch material, and an anatomical structure such as an AV valve annulus, vena cava or pulmonary vein, in which conduction velocity is slower than normal, and from which concealed entrainment may be demonstrated [7-8]. This isthmus is not only critical to the development of reentry, but in a manner similar to the TV-IVC isthmus in AFL, its ablated will interrupt and cure the AT [7-8].

Atrial tachycardia may also be focal in origin [47-48]. Focal AT may be due to abnormal automaticity or triggered activity arising from an area of scar tissue or from the pulmonary veins or coronary sinus. Because of its electrophysiologic mechanism, focal AT cannot be entrained and may not be terminated by rapid overdrive atrial pacing. However, in many cases focal AT can be cured by localized ablation [48]. It has also been recently recognized that focal AT may precipitate or mimic AFIB, in which case AFIB may actually be cured by localized ablation [49-50].

Atrial fibrillation is characterized by a rapid, irregular atrial rhythm at a rate of greater than 350 beats per minute, resulting in the absence of distinct P waves an irregularly, irregular ventricular response on ECG. Atrial fibrillation is in most cases due to multiple reentrant wavelets simultaneously propagating throughout the right and left atrium [3-4]. These multiple reentrant circuits appear to be both functionally and anatomically determined [3-4]. Studies in both animals and humans have suggested that the multiple reentrant circuits responsible for AFIB may develop as a result of abnormal shortening and dispersion of atrial refractory period and abnormal slowing of atrial conduction velocity [51-55]. Such atrial electrophysiologic abnormalities may result from underlying valvular or myocardial dysfunction or systemic hypertension causing atrial stretch and enlargement, ischemia, or simply aging alone, and may be aggravated in the post-operative period by hemodynamic instability, increased sympathetic and vagal nervous system activity, pericardial inflammation, hypoxia, or electrolyte disturbances. Due to the fact that the reentrant circuits are predominately functionally determined, AFIB cannot be entrained nor terminated by rapid overdrive atrial pacing. Atrial fibrillation may be converted and suppressed by antiarrhythmic drugs, the most effective being those which prolong atrial refractoriness in a use-dependent manner. However, since AFIB involves multiple reentrant circuits, its cure requires creation of extensive linear lesions, either surgically or by catheter ablation, between all or the majority of anatomical structures in the right and left atria in order to interrupt all potential reentrant circuits [56-57].

3. Experimental Animal Models of Atrial Flutter and Atrial Tachycardia

Spontaneous atrial flutter or tachycardia occur only rarely in animals [58]. Therefore, a number of experimental animal models have been developed in order to study the electrophysiologic mechanisms of AFL and AT, and their response to antiarrhythmic drugs and other curative interventions.

One of the earliest in vivo models of sustained, reentrant AFL was that of the canine inter-caval crush model studied by Rosenbleuth and Garcia-Ramos [17]. This model involved reentry around an anatomical obstacle created by crushing the inter-caval region. The resultant AFL induced by rapid atrial pacing, was found to have a fully excitable gap similar to that in human atrial flutter. In this model, AFL could be terminated by drugs such as the antihistaminic agent clemizole, which prolonged atrial refractory period. However, detailed activation mapping studies were not been done in this model by the original investigators. Therefore, it is unknown if the reentry circuit in the inter-caval crush model also utilized the TV-IVC isthmus, as it does in human AFL, or if it was confined to the right atrial posterior wall around the inter-caval crush. Subsequently, alternative in-vivo experimental canine models, such as the tricuspid ring and right atrial crush-injury models, were developed in an attempt to better characterize AFL and other reentrant AT.

The canine right atrial tricuspid ring model of atrial flutter is characterized by a single, anatomically determined reentry circuit, with a partially excitable gap [18-19]. In this model, through a right thoracotomy and pericardiotomy, a branching Y-shaped incision is made in the right atrium, consisting of an inter-caval incision from superior to inferior vena cava, and a right atrial incision connected to the inter-caval incision about one-third of the way up from the inferior vena cava (Figure 1).

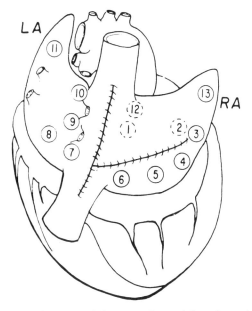

Figure 1. Schematic diagram of the posterior atrial surfaces indicating the location of the Y-incision used to create atrial flutter due to reentry in the supra-annular tissue around the tricuspid valve ring. Note the Y-incision consists of a vertical incision in the inter-caval region and a connecting horizontal incision extending towards the right atrial appendage in the right atrial free wall. Reproduced with permission from reference 17.

Following creation of the Y-incision AFL is then induced by rapid atrial pacing. The cycle length of AFL in this model ranges from 140-170 msec. Classical entrainment criteria can be demonstrated, confirming its reentrant mechanism. Activation mapping of the right atrium (Figure 2) has shown that the reentry circuit is involves the atrial tissue above the tricuspid valve annulus [59], similar to that of human type 1 AFL. However, the canine tricuspid ring model of AFL differs from human type 1 AFL in several respects. First, the Y-incision in this model confines the reentry circuit to the supra-annular atrial tissue, preventing any reentrant wavefront moving cephalad in the inter-atrial septum from propagating over the right atrial free wall or around the crista terminalis, as occurs in human type 1 AFL. Secondly, studies in this model have characterized the reentry circuit as having only a partially excitable gap, in contrast to human type 1 AFL where there is a fully excitable gap [18-19]. Thus, while the tricuspid ring model of AFL is an excellent model for studying reentrant atrial arrhythmias, it may not be ideally suited for the study of human type 1 AFL because its electrophysiologic characteristics differ somewhat. However, because it is a surgically

6

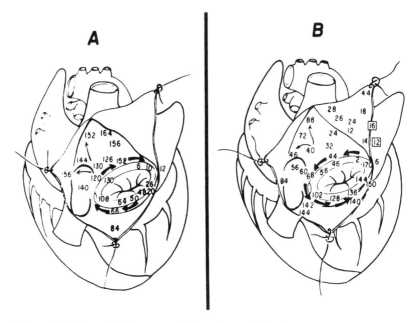

Figure 2. Schematic diagrams of the endocardial activation sequences during clockwise (A) and counter-clockwise (B) atrial flutter induced in the Y-incision or tricuspid ring model. The endocardial surface of the right atrium is viewed through the Y-incision or tricuspid ring model. The endocardial surface of the right atrium is viewed through the Y-incision. Reproduced with permission from reference 17.

created model with anatomical obstacles, its characteristics may have relevance to some AT seen after surgery for congenital heart disease. In addition, studies in this model have provided significant insight into the mechanisms of termination of AFL. For example, the mechanisms of spontaneous and pharmacological termination of reentry have been extensively studied in this model, demonstrating the role of both cycle length oscillation and failure of lateral boundaries of the reentry circuit as mechanisms responsible for arrhythmia termination [60-62].

The canine right atrial crush-injury model of AFL is characterized by a single, anatomically determined reentry circuit, with a fully excitable gap, similar to that of human type 1 atrial flutter [20-21]. To create this model, a linear crush-injury, approximately 1.5 to 2.5 cm long is made by placing a surgical clamp on the right atrial free wall, parallel to and approximately 1.5 cm above the tricuspid annulus (Figure 3).

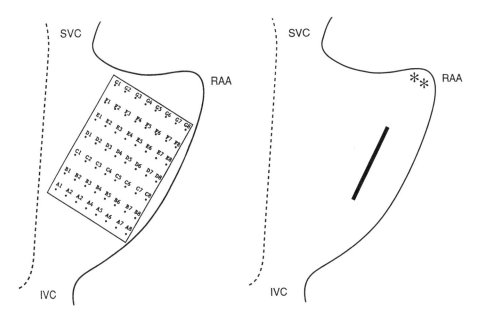

Figure 3. Schematic diagrams of the crush-injury and the electrode mapping plaque in the canine crush-injury model of AFL. (A) A high-density electrode plaque is sutured on the epicardial surface of the right atrial free wall for activation mapping. Then plaque dimensions measured 4.5 X 3.5 cm. (B) Thecrush-injury (solid line) is made on the right atrial free wall, parallel to and approximately 1.5 cm above the tricuspid valve annulus, extending from the base of the right atrial appendage posteriorly toward the inter-caval zone. Crush-injury length ranged from 1.5 to 2.5 cm and width approximately 3-4 mm. IVC = inferior vena cava, RAA = right atrial appendage, SVC = superior vena cava, TV = tricuspid valve. * = location of pacing electrodes.

Following the crush-injury AFL is induced by rapid atrial pacing in over 90% of animals [20-21]. The cycle length of AFL induced in this model ranges from 120-180 msec. Classical entrainment criteria can be demonstrated, confirming its reentrant mechanism. Activation mapping has shown that the reentry circuit encircles the right atrial crush-injury (Figure 4).

8

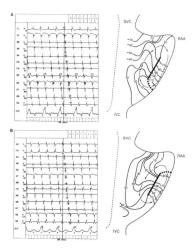

Figure 4. Electrograms and activation patterns during sustained atrial flutter in the canine right atrial crush-injury model. Left panel: Sequential electrograms from around the reentrant circuit and surface ECG lead a VF are shown during episodes of counterclockwise (A) and clockwise (B) atrial flutter in the canine right atrial crush-injury model. Right panel: Right atrial activation maps are shown demonstrating counterclockwise (A) and clockwise (B) activation patterns (as viewed from anterior to the heart) during the same episodes of atrial flutter shown in the left panel. Abbreviations same as in Figure 3. Dotted activation line separates earliest and latest activation times during atrial flutter on activation map. On electrogram recordings the solid vertical line represents a reference mark at the onset of the P wave in the surface ECG. Cross-hairs following the reference line represent computer assigned local activation times for each atrial electrogram.

Furthermore, the crush-injury behaves as an anatomical obstacle, along which double-potentials may be recorded during AFL, and during atrial pacing on either side of the crush-injury at a slow rate [21]. Between the crush-injury and the tricuspid valve annulus is an isthmus of atrial tissue with relatively slow conduction velocity compared to other atrial tissue in the reentry circuit. The induction of AFL in this model results from the development of conduction block in the more slowly conducting isthmus between the crush-injury and tricuspid valve annulus [20,63-64]. Pharmacological termination of AFL in this model (Figure 5) has been shown to be due to development of conduction block in this isthmus as well [63-64].

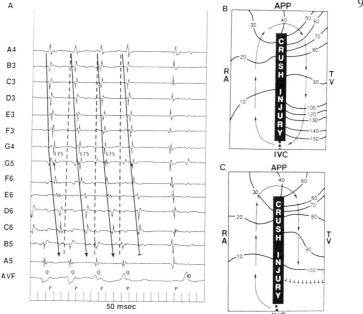

Figure 5. Activation patterns and electrogram recordings during termination of atrial flutter by intravenous infusion of the class 3 antiarrhythmic drug dofetilide. (A) Epicardial electrograms from around the crush-injury during the last few beats of atrial flutter demonstrating abrupt termination without cycle length oscillation, as a result of failure of wavefront propagation between electrodes B5 and A5. (B) An activation map from mapping the plaque only during this same episode of atrial flutter demonstrates the reentrant circuit around the crush-injury during the next-to-last beat prior to termination. (C) An activation map from mapping the plaque only during the last beat of atrial flutter demonstrates termination by abrupt failure of wavefront propagation below the posterior end of the crush-injury. —| = site of conduction block. APP = right atrial appendage, IVC = inferior vena cava, RA = right atrium, TV = tricuspid valve annulus.

Furthermore, termination of AFL may occur either abruptly without cycle length oscillation, or following premature eccentric activation of the reentry circuit presumably due to failure of its lateral boundaries [20,63-64]. Pharmacological termination of AFL in this model is associated with prolongation of atrial wavelength and a decrease in excitable gap, but calculations performed during studies comparing the effects of the class 1 and 3 antiarrhythmic drugs suggest that impulse propagation ultimately fails due to a reduced safety factor for conduction in the area of slow conduction, rather than complete elimination of the excitable gap [63-64]. Thus, since the electrophysiologic characteristics of the canine crush-injury model of AFL are in many ways similar to those of human type 1 AFL, it is an appropriate model to study potential mechanisms and treatment. In fact, studies in the canine crush-injury model [63-66] have shown that class 3 antiarrhythmic drugs (e.g. sotalol, dofetilide, n-acetylprocainamide) that prolong atrial refractory period and wavelength and reduce dispersion of refractoriness, are more effective in terminating and preventing reinduction of AFL than the class 1 antiarrhythmic drugs (e.g. quinidine, lidocaine, recainam). Clinical studies have subsequently shown this to be true in human type 1 AFL as well, with class 3 drugs such as ibutilide achieving higher conversion rates than those observed with the class 1 antiarrhythmic drugs such as quinidine [67]. Since the canine crush-injury model of AFL is created by placing a surgical lesion in the right atrium its mechanism and electrophysiologic characteristics are also similar to those of post-operative "scar tachycardia" in humans, making it an appropriate model for the study of these arrhythmias as well [15,24].

The canine sterile pericarditis model of AFL, in contrast to those described above, is characterized by a functionally determined reentry circuit that has a regionally variable (i.e. partial to full) excitable gap [22-23]. In this model, through a right thoracotomy and pericardiotomy, sterile talcum powder is dusted onto the epicardial surfaces of the right and left atria, which are then covered with a single layer of gauze. The pericardium and chest are then closed and the animal is allowed to fully recover post-operatively. For several days following surgery, sustained AFL can then be induced by rapid atrial pacing from implanted atrial epicardial electrodes. Following rapid atrial pacing, a brief period of AFIB often proceeds the development of a stable AFL in this model. At 24-hours following surgery up to 70-80% of animals have inducible AFL, however the inducibility of AFL declines over time to less than 50% of animals after seven days. The cycle length of induced AFL ranges from 125-155 msec. Right atrial epicardial activation mapping studies (Figure 6) have shown that the induction of AFL by rapid atrial pacing results from development of a line of conduction block that is usually contiguous with an anatomical structure such as the tricuspid valve annulus [68-70]. Reentry is then established around a functional line of block at the center of the reentry circuit that stabilizes and remains fixed during any individual episode of AFL [68-70]. Double potentials, like those observed in human type 1 AFL, can be recorded along these functional lines of block during AFL [69]. However, since the lines of conduction block responsible for the induction and

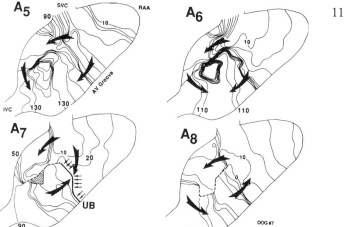

Figure 6: Posterior right atrial epicardial activation patterns during induction of atrial flutter in the canine sterile pericarditis model. Note during the onset of atrial flutter after rapid atrial pacing that areas of slow conduction develop (tachycardia beats A5-A6) as indicated by closely spaced activation isochrones, followed by development of unidirectional block in an area of slow conduction contiguous with the tricuspid valve nnulus (tachycardia beat A7), followed by development of stable reentry around a fixed functional line of block at the center of the reentry circuit (tachycardia beta A8). Reproduced with permission from reference 69.

maintenance of AFL in the sterile pericarditis model are functionally determined, their location may vary significantly between animals and from one episode of AFL to another [69], in contrast to human type 1 AFL or the anatomical lesion models of AFL in which the lines of conduction block are constant. Furthermore, unlike human type 1 AFL, pharmacological conversion rates of AFL in the sterile pericarditis model are similar between the class 1 and 3 antiarrhythmic drugs. Activation mapping studies during pharmacological termination of AFL in the sterile pericarditis model revealed that the class 1 and 3 antiarrhythmic drugs uniformly caused further slowing of conduction and block in areas of preexisting slow conduction in the reentrant circuit [69]. Thus, regardless of their differing effects on wavelength and excitable gap, the class 1 and 3 antiarrhythmic drugs appear to terminate AFL in this model by reducing the safety factor for conduction in the area of slow conduction in the reentrant circuit [69]. Thus, the electrophysiologic characteristics of the canine sterile pericarditis model of AFL appear to be more similar to those of human type 2 AFL than to type 1 AFL.

The canine right atrial enlargement model of AFL is characterized by a functionally determined reentry circuit that is very similar to that of the sterile pericarditis model [24-25]. In this model, through a thoracotomy the chorda tendineae of the anterior and septal tricuspid valve leaflets are cut to produce tricuspid valve regurgitation, which is enhanced post-operatively by inflating a hydraulic occluder placed around the main pulmonary artery at the time of surgery in order to produce pulmonary artery stenosis. After 4-8 weeks, during which significant right atrial enlargement occurs, sustained atrial flutter can be induced in the majority of animals by rapid atrial pacing. Activation mapping studies have been done in this model of AFL in the isolated, Langendorf perfused heart, using an endocardial egg-shaped multi-electrode plaque, inserted through the right ventricle and tricuspid valve into the right atrium [24-25]. The induction and maintenance of AFL (Figure 7) is dependent on

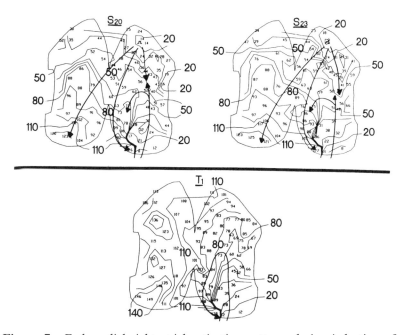

Figure 7. Endocardial right atrial activation patterns during induction of atrial flutter. Note that during rapid atrial pacing a functional line of block develops in the low posterior right atrium contiguous with the tricuspid valve annulus (pacing beats S20-S23), following which stable reentry develops around a fixed functional line of block (tachycardia beat T1). Reproduced with permission from reference 25.

development of functional lines of block, in a manner very similar to that observed in the sterile pericarditis model of AFL [24-25]. Class 3 antiarrhythmic drugs effectively slow and terminate AFL in this model, as seen in other animal models of AFL and human type 1 AFL. [25,71]. However, like the sterile pericarditis model of AFL, the right atrial enlargement model has electrophysiologic characteristics that are more similar to those of human type 2 AFL than to type 1 AFL.

Aconitine induced focal AT is actually one of the earliest animal models of atrial tachycardia developed, and it is characterized by rapid, sometimes irregular atrial depolarization [72]. In this model, a small quantity of aconitine is placed on the atrial epicardial surface, causing rapid focal discharges of the underlying atrial tissue. Because of its focal nature, aconitine induced focal AT cannot be entrained, nor is it inducible or terminated by rapid atrial pacing. Since the resulting arrhythmia is most likely due to triggered automaticity and not reentry, its mechanism may be similar to that of focal AT seen in humans. When very fast, aconitine induced focal AT may resemble AFIB, which may have relevance to the recently recognized phenomenon of focal AFIB caused by an underlying AT in humans [49-50].

4. Experimental Animal Models of Atrial Fibrillation

Several experimental models of atrial fibrillation have been recently developed including the vagally mediated AFIB model in the dog [26-27] and the rapid atrial pacing-induced AFIB model in the goat [28-29].

The vagally mediated AFIB model in the dog is produced by high-frequency stimulation of the vagus nerve, which results in marked shortening and dispersion of atrial refractoriness [26,27]. During vagal stimulation AFIB can be easily induced by rapid atrial pacing [26-27]. Atrial fibrillation is then sustained as long as vagal stimulation is maintained. Mapping of atrial fibrillation in this model demonstrates the presence of multiple wavelets or reentrant circuits simultaneously activating the right and left atria, in a pattern consistent with that observed during human atrial fibrillation. In this model, antiarrhythmic drugs which prolong atrial refractory period (e.g. the class 1c and 3 antiarrhythmic drugs) have been shown to terminate AFIB by prolonging atrial wavelength, and reducing the number of circulating reentrant wavelets until reentrant activation is eventually interrupted due to conduction block. Furthermore, antiarrhythmic drugs that prolong atrial refractory period in a use-dependent manner (e.g. the class 1c drugs flecainide and propafenone) are particularly effective in terminating AFIB, an observation which has also been made in humans. The underlying mechanism of this model of AFIB may be particularly relevant to AFIB occurring in the post-operative setting where vagal tone may be high.

The rapid atrial pacing-induced model of AFIB in the goat (Figure 8) is produced by repeatedly burst pacing the atrium, using an implantable custom designed automatic atrial fibrillator (Medtronic, Inc.) programmed to pace the atrium with a 1-second burst of stimuli at a cycle length of 20 msec at four times diastolic threshold whenever sinus rhythm is detected, until AFIB becomes sustained [28-29]. In this model, AFIB typically becomes sustained after several days of repeated induction by burst pacing. Studies in this model have shown that sustained rapid atrial pacing or

14

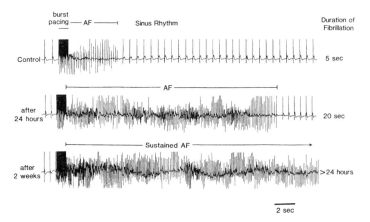

Figure 8. Atrial electrogram recordings in the rapid atrial pacing model of atrial fibrillation in the goat. Note that following increasingly prolonged periods of rapid atrial pacing atrial fibrillation becomes more prolonged and eventually sustained, due to shortening of atrial refractory period and electrical remodeling. Reproduced with permission from reference 28.

sustained AFIB markedly shortens atrial refractory period to an average of 95±20 msec from an average of 146±19 msec at baseline, which results in significant shortening of atrial wavelength and increased vulnerability to AFIB (i.e. electrical remodeling). It has also been demonstrated in this model that rapid atrial pacing for prolonged periods or prolonged episodes of AFIB lead to ultrastructural damage in atrial myocytes, including damage to the mitochondria and sarcoplasmic reticulum. Furthermore reversion of AFIB to sinus rhythm is associated with rapid recovery of the abnormally shortened refractory period in the atria. Studies in this model have shown that pretreatment with calcium channel blockers such as verapamil prevents electrical remodeling during rapid atrial pacing. Interestingly, pretreatment of humans with oral calcium channel blocking drugs prior to electrical cardioversion of AFIB also reduces short-term recurrence rates, which may be due in part to prevention of electrical remodeling [73]. Extensive investigation of this rapid atrial pacing-induced model of AFIB in the goat is currently underway in order better delineate its mechanisms and causes. Atrial fibrillation may also be induced in the canine in a similar manner to that produced in the goat [74]. This model may have significant relevance to the initiation and maintenance of AFIB in humans in the post-operative setting, especially those with a history of AFIB.

Other less commonly used experimental models of AFIB have been described, including induction of AFIB by continuous infusion of theophylline in the sheep, which shortens atrial refractory period and wavelength, increasing atrial vulnerability [75]. Atrial fibrillation may also be induced in the canine sterile pericarditis and right atrial enlargement models [22-25], and in a small percentage of canines without chronic atrial pacing [76].

5. Conclusion

Studies in these numerous animal models of atrial arrhythmias have significantly enhanced our understanding of the electrophysiologic characteristics of atrial flutter, atrial tachycardia and atrial fibrillation in humans. Although extrapolation of observations made in animal models of arrhythmias to human arrhythmias has some limitations, each of the models described in this chapter has important similarities to specific human atrial arrhythmias. Thus, the use of experimental arrhythmia models remains an important tool for understanding the mechanisms of cardiac arrhythmias and for the development of new methods for their effective treatment.

References

1.   Michelson EL, Morganroth J, MacVaugh H. Postoperative arrhythmias after coronary artery and cardiac valvular surgery detected by long-term electrocardiographic monitoring Am Heart T 1982;104:442-448.
2.   Yousif H, Davies G, Oakley CM. Peri-operative supraventricular arrhythmias in coronary artery bypass graft surgery. Int J Cardiol 1990;26:313-318.
3.   Cox JL, Canavan TE, Scheussler RB, et.al. The surgical treatment of atrial fibrillation. II. Intraoperative electrophysiologic mapping and description of the basis of atrial flutter and atrial fibrillation. J Thorac Cardiovasc Surg 1991;101:406-426.
4.   Jalife J, Berenfeld O, Skanes A, Mandapati R. Mechanism of atrial fibrillation: Mother rotors or multiple daughter wavelets or both. J Cardiovasc Electrophysiol 1998;9:S2-S12.
5.   Disertori M, Inama G, Vergara G, Guanerio M, Del Favero A, Furlanello F. Evidence of a reentry circuit in the common type of atrial flutter in man. Circulation 1963;67:434-440.
6.   Waldo AL, MacLean WAH, Karp RB, Kouchoukos NT, James TN. Entrainment and interruption of atrial flutter with atrial pacing: Studies in man following open-heart surgery. Circulation 1997;56:737-745.
7.   Lesh MD, Kalman JM, Saxon LA, Dorostkar PE. Electrophysiology of "incisional" reentrant atrial tachycardia complicating surgery for congenital heart disease. Pacing Clin Electrophysiol 1997;20:2107-2111.
8.   Kalman JM, VenHare GF, Olgin JE, Saxon LA, Stark SI, Lesh MD. Ablation of "incisional' reentrant atrial tachycardia complicating surgery for congenital heart disease. Use of entrainment to define a critical isthmus of conduction. Circulation 1996;93:502-512.
9.   Kuck KH, Ernst S, Cappato R, Braun E, et.al. Nonfluoroscopic mapping of atrial fibrillation. J Cardiovasc Electrophysiol 1998;9:S57-S62.
10.   Pitschner HF, Berkovic A, Grumbrecht S, Neuzner J. Multielectrode basket catheter mapping for human atrial fibrillation. J Cardiovasc Electrophysiol 1998;9:S48-S56.
11.   Cosio FG, Arribas F, Lopez-Gil M, Palacios J. Atrial flutter mapping or ablation I. Studying atrial flutter mechanisms by mapping and entrainment. Pacing Clin Electrophysiol 1996;19:841-853.
12.   Cosio FG, Goicolea A, Lopez-Gil M, Arribal S, Barroso JL. Atrial endocardial mapping in the rare form of atrial flutter. Am J Cardiol 1990;66:715-720.
13.   Kottkamp H, Hindricks G, Breithardt G, Borgreffe M. Three-dimensional electromagnetic catheter technology: Electroanatomical mapping of the right atrium and ablation of ectopic atrial tachycardia. J Cardiovasc Electrophysiol 1997;8:1332-1337.
14.   Feld GK: Catheter Ablation for the Treatment of Atrial Tachycardias. Prog Cardiovas Dis 38:205-224,1995.

15. Konigs KT, Kirchhof CJ Smeets JR, Wellens HJ, Penn OC Allessie MA. High density mapping of electrically induced atrial fibrillation in humans. Circulation 1994;89:1665-1680.

16. Klein GJ, Guiraudon GM, Sharma AD, Milstein S. Demonstration of macroreentry and feasibility of operative therapy in the common type of atrial flutter. Am J Cardiol 1986;57:587-591.

17. Rosenbleuth A, Garcia-Ramos J. Studies of artificial obstacles on experimental auricular flutter. Am Heart J 1947;33:677-684.

18. Frame LH, Page RL, Hoffman BG. Atrial re-entry around an anatomic barrier with a partially excitable gap. A canine model of atrial flutter. Circ Res 1986;58:495-511.

19. Frame LH. The tricuspid ring model of atrial flutter. In: Waldo AL, Touboul P, (eds). "Atrial Flutter: Advances in Mechanisms and Management." Armonk, NY, Futura Publishing Co., 1996, pp 159-172.

20. Feld GK, Shahandeh-Rad F. Activation patterns in experimental canine atrial flutter produced by right atrial crush-injury. J Am Coll Cardiol 1992;20:441-451.

21. Feld GK, Shehandeh-Rad F. Mechanism of double potentials recorded during sustained atrial flutter in the canine right atrial crush-injury model. Circulation 1992;86:628-641.

22. Pagé PL, Plumb VJ, Okumura K, Waldo L. A new animal model of atrial flutter. J Am Coll Cardiol 1986;8:872-879.

23. Okumura K, Plumb VJ, Pagé PL, Waldo AL. Atrial activation sequence during atrial flutter in the canine pericarditis model and its effects on the polarity of the flutter wave in the electrocardiogram. J Am Coll Cardiol 1991;17:509-518.

24. Boyden PA. Activation sequence during atrial flutter in dogs with surgically-induced right atrial enlargement. I: Observations during sustained rhythms. Circ Res 1988;62:596-607.

25. Boyden PA. Studies in animal models of atrial flutter. Tricuspid regurgitation model. In: Waldo AL, Touboul P, (eds). "Atrial Flutter: Advances in Mechanisms and Management." Armonk, NY, Futura Publishing Co., 1996, pp 137-157.

26. Wang Z, Page P, Nattel S. Mechanism of flecainide's antiarrhythmic action in experimental atrial fibrillation. Circ Res 1992;71:271-287.

27. Wang J, Bourne GW, Wang Z, Villemaire C, Talajic M, Nattel S. Comparative mechanisms of drug action in experimental atrial fibrillation. Importance of use-dependent effects on refractoriness. Circulation 1993;88:1030-1044.

28. Wijffels MC, Kirchhof CJ, Dorland R, Allessie MA. Atrial fibrillation begets atrial fibrillation. A study in awake chronically instrumented goats. Circulation 1995;92:1954-1968.

29. Wijffels MC, Kirchhof CJ, Dorland R, Power J, Allessie MA. Electrical remodeling due to atrial fibrillation in chronically instrumented conscious goats: Roles of neurohumoral changes, ischemia, atrial stretch, and high rate of electrical activation. Circulation 1997;96:3710-3720.

30. Waldo AL. Transient entrainment of atrial flutter. In: Waldo AL, Touboul P, (eds). "Atrial Flutter: Advances in Mechanisms and Management." Armonk, NY, Futura Publishing Co., 1996, pp 241-257.

31. Inoue H, Matsuo H, Takayangi K, Murao S: Clinical and experimental studies of the effects of atrial extrastimulation and rapid pacing on atrial flutter cycle. Am J Cardiol 1981;48:623-631.

32. Feld GK, Fleck RP, Chen PS, Boyce K, Bahnson TD, Stein JB, Calisi CM, Ibarra M. Radiofrequency catheter ablation for the treatment of human type 1 atrial flutter. Identification of a critical zone in the reentrant circuit by endocardial mapping techniques. Circulation 1992;86:1233-1240.

33. Cosio RG, López-Gil M, Goicolea A, Arribas F, Barroso JL. Radiofrequency ablation of the inferior vena cava-tricuspid valve isthmus in common atrial flutter. Am J Cardiol 1993;71:705-709.

34. Olshansky B, Okumura K, Hess PG, Waldo AL. Demonstration of an area of slow conduction in human atrial flutter. J Am Coll Cardiol 1990;16:1639-1648.

35. Feld GK, Mollerus M, Birgersdotter-Green U, Fujimura O, Bahnson T, Boyce K, Rahme M. Conduction velocity in the tricuspid valve - inferior vena cava isthmus is slower in patients with a history of atrial flutter compared to those without atrial flutter. J Cardiovasc Electrophysiol 8:1338-1348, 1997.

36. Olgin JE, Kalman JM, Saxon LA, Lee RJ, Lesh MD. Mechanisms of initiation of atrial flutter in humans: Site of unidirectional block and direction of rotation. J Am Coll Cardiol 1997;29:376-384.

37. Ching TT, Chen SA Chiang CE, et.al. Characterization of low right atrial isthmus as the slow

conduction zone and pharmacological target in typical atrial flutter. Circulation 1997;96:2601-2611.

38. Tai CT, Chan SA, Feng AN, Yu WC, Chen YJ, Chng MS. Electropharmacological effects of class 1 and 3 antiarrhythmic drugs on typical atrial flutter: Insights into mechanism of termination. Circulation 1998;97:1335-1345.

39. Cosio FG, Arribas F, Palacios J, Tascon J, Lopez-Gil M. Fragmented electrograms and continuous electrical activity in atrial flutter. Am J Cardiol 19986;57:1309-1314.

40. Cosio FG, Arribus F, Barbero JM, Kallmeyer C, Goicolea A. Validation of double spike electrograms as markers of conduction delay or block in atrial flutter. Am J Cardiol 1988;61:775-780.

41. Olshansky B, Okumura K, Henthorn RW, Waldo AL. Characterization of double potentials in human atrial flutter: Studies during transient entrainment. J Am Coll Cardiol 1990;15:833-841.

42. Olgin JE, Kalman JM, Fizpatrick AP, Lesh MD. Role of right atrial endocardial structures as barriers to conduction during human type 1 atrial flutter. Activation and entrainment mapping guided by intracardiac echocardiography. Circulation 1995;92:1839-1848.

43. Olgin JE, Kalman JM, Lesh MD. Conduction barriers in human atrial flutter: Correlation of electrophysiology and anatomy. J Cardiovasc Electrophysiol 1996;7:1112-1126.

44. Kalman, JM, Olgin JE, Saxon LA, Fischer WG, Lee RJ, Lesh MD. Activation and entrainment mapping defines the tricuspid annulus as the anterior barrier in typical atrial flutter. Circulation 1996;94:398-406.

45. Wells JL Jr, MacLean WAH, James TN, Waldo AL. Characterization of atrial flutter: Studies in man after open-heart surgery using fixed atrial electrodes. Circulation 1979;60:665-673.

46. Waldo AL, Plumb VJ, Arciniegas JG, et.al. Observations on the mechanism of atrial flutter. In Surawicz B (ed): Tachycardias. The Hague, Martinus-Nijhoff, 1984, p 213.

47. Chen SA, Tai CT, Chiang CE, Ding YA, Chang MS. Focal atrial tachycardia: Reanalysis of the clinical and electrophysiological characteristics and prediction of successful radiofrequency ablation. J Cardiovasc Electrophysiol 1998;9:355-365.

48. Kay GN, Chong F, Epstein AE, Dailey SM, Plumb VJ. Radiofrequency ablation for treatment of primary atrial tachycardia. J Am Coll Cardiol 1993;21:901-909.

49. Haissaguerre M, Gensel L, Fischer B, LeMetayer P, Poquet F, Marcus FL, Clementy J. Successful catheter ablation of atrial fibrillation. J Cardiovasc Electrophysiol 1994;5:1045-1052

50. Jais P, Haissaguerre M, Shah DC, Chouairi S, Gencel L, Hocini M, Clementy J. A focal source of atrial fibrillation treated by discrete radiofrequency ablation. Circulation 1997;95:572-576.

51. Rensma PL, Allessie MA, Lammers WJFP, Bonke FIM, Schalij MJ. Length of excitation wave and susceptibility to reentrant atrial arrhythmias in normal conscious dogs. Circ Res 1988;62:395-410.

52. Wang Z, Feng J, Nattel S. Idiopathic atrial fibrillation in dogs: Electrophysiological determinants and mechanisms of antiarrhythmic action of flecainide. J Am Coll Cardiol 1995;26:277-286.

53. Rahme MM, Leistad E, Cotter B, Simu S, Bahnson TD, Feld GK. Maintenance of atrial fibrillation: Dependence on the duration and dispersion of atrial refractoriness (abstract). Pacing Clin Electrophysiol 1988;21:863.

54. Ramdat Misier AR, Opthof T, van Hemel NM, et.al. Increased dispersion of refractoriness in patients with idiopathic paroxysmal atrial fibrillation. J Am Coll Cardiol 1992;19:1531-1535.

55. Kumagai K, Akimitsu S, Kawahira K, et.al. Electrophysiological properties in chronic lone atrial fibrillation. Circulation 1991;84:1662-1668.

56. Cox JL, Boineau JP, Schuessler RB, et al: Five-year experience with Maze procedure for atrial fibrillation. Ann Thorac Surg 1993:56:814-824.

57. Haissaguerre M, Jais P, Shah DC, Gencel L, Pradeau v, Garrigues S, Chouairi S, Hocini M, Le Metayer P, Roudaut R, Clementy J. Right and left atrial radiofrequency catheter therapy of paroxysmal atrial fibrillation. J Cardiovasc Electrophysiol. 1996;7:1132-1144.

58. Biouneau JP, Schuessler RB, Mooney CR, et.al. Natural and evoked atrial flutter due to circus movement in dogs: Role of abnormal atrial pathways, slow conduction, non-uniform refractory period distribution and premature beats. Am J Cardiol 1980;45:1167-1181.

59. Frame LH, Page RL, Boyden PA, et.al. Circus movement in the canine atrium around the tricuspid

18

ring during experimental atria flutter and during reentry in vivo. Circulation 1987;76:1155-1175.

60.   Frame LH, Simson MB. Oscillations of conduction, action potential duration and refractoriness: A mechanism for spontaneous termination or reentrant tachycardias. Circulation 1988;78:1277-1287.

61.   Boyden P, Graziano H. Activation mapping of reentry around an anatomical barrier in the canine atrium: Observations during the action of the class III agent, d-sotalol. J Cardiovasc Electrophysiol 1993;4:266-279.

62.   Pinto J, Graziano J, Boyden P. Endocardial mapping of reentry around an anatomical barrier in the canine right atrium: Observations during the action of the class IC agent, flecainide. J Cardiovasc Electrophysiol 1993;4:672-685.

63.   Feld GK: Characteristics of the canine crush-injury model of atrial flutter. In: Atrial Flutter: Advances in Mechanisms and Management. Waldo AL, Touboul P, eds; Futura Publishing Co., Armonk, NY, 1996, pp 193-217.

64.   Cha YM, Wales A, Wolf P, Shahrokni S, Sawhney N, Feld GK. Electrophysiologic effects of the new class 3 antiarrhythmic drug dofetilide compared to the class 1a antiarrhythmic drug quinidine in experimental canine atrial flutter: Role of dispersion of refractoriness in antiarrhythmic efficacy. J Cardiovasc Electrophysiol 7:809-827, 1996.

65.   Feld GK, Venkatesh N, Singh BN. Pharmacologic conversion and suppression of experimental canine atrial flutter. Differing effects of D-sotalol, quinidine and lidocaine and the significance of changes in refractoriness and conduction. Circulation 74(1):197-204, 1986.

66.   Feld GK, Venkatesh N, Singh BN: Effects of N-acetylprocainamide and recainam in experimental canine atrial flutter: Significance of the changes in refractoriness and conduction velocity in the conversion and suppression of atrial flutter. J Cardiovasc Phar 11:573-580, 1988.

67.   Stambler BS, Wood MA, Ellenbogen KA. Antiarrhythmic actions of intravenous ibutilide compared with procainamide during human atrial flutter and atrial fibrillation: Electrophysiological determinants of enhanced conversion efficacy. Circulation 1997;96:4298-4306.

68.   Shimizu A, Nozaki A, Rudy Y, Waldo AL. Onset of induced atrial flutter in the canine pericarditis model. J Am Coll Cardiol 1991;17:1223-1234.

69.   Waldo AL. The canine sterile pericarditis model of atrial flutter. In: Atrial Flutter: Advances in Mechanisms and Management. Waldo AL, Touboul P, eds; Futura Publishing Co., Armonk, NY, 1996, pp 173-192.

70.   Schöels W, Gough WB, Restive M, El-Sherif N. Circus movement atrial flutter in the canine sterile pericarditis model. Activation patterns during initiation, termination and sustained re-entry in vivo. Circ Res 1990;67:35-50.

71.   Boyden, PA. Effects of pharmacologic agents on induced atrial flutter in dogs with right atrial enlargement. J Cardiovasc Pharm 1986;8:170-177.

72.   Brown BB, Acheson GH. Aconitine induced auricular arrhythmias and their relation to circus movement and flutter. Circulation 1952;6:529.

73.   Tieleman, RG, Van Gelder, IC, Crijns, HJG, De Kam, PJ, Van Den Berg, MP, Haaksma, J, Van Der Woude, HJ, Allessie, MA. Early recurrences of atrial fibrillation after electrical cardioversion: A result of fibrillation induced electrical remodeling of the atria? J Am Coll Cardiol 1998;31:167-73.

74.   Arzbaecher R, Gemperline J, Haklin M, Bucemi P. Rapid drug infusion for termination of atrial fibrillation in an experimental model. Pacing Clin Electrophysiol 1998;21:288-291.

75.   Fieguth HG, Wahlers T, Borst HG. Inhibition of atrial fibrillation by pulmonary vein isolation and auricular resection – Experimental study in a sheep model. Europ J Cardio Thorac Surg 1997;11:714-721.

76.   Wang Z, Feng J, Nattel S. Idiopathic atrial fibrillation in dogs: Electrophysiologic determinants and mechanisms of antiarrhythmic action of flecainide. J Am Coll Cardiol 1995;26:277-286.

2 UNDERSTANDING THE PATHOPHYSIOLOGY OF ATRIAL FIBRILLATION FROM CLINICAL OBSERVATIONS

Scott E. Mattson, MD and Leonard I. Ganz,MD, Allegheny General Hospital, Pittsburgh, PA

1. Introduction

Atrial fibrillation (AF) is the most commonly encountered sustained arrhythmia in man [1]. A number of conditions are associated with the development of AF, including cardiac surgery. The incidence of AF after cardiac surgery, however, far exceeds the incidence of AF in the general population, or in patients with ischemic heart disease [2,3,4]. In this chapter, anatomic and pathophysiologic factors associated with AF will be explored, with particular consideration to those relevant to cardiac surgery.

Atrial fibrillation occurs relatively frequently in the general population, increasing in prevalence with advancing age (Figure 1) [5], and usually presents in association with hypertension and/or structural cardiac diseases [6,7]. Conversely, AF is uncommon in patients with structurally normal hearts [8]. Table 1 demonstrates the risk of AF associated with hypertension, valvular heart disease, prior myocardial infarction and congestive heart failure [6]. As the majority of patients undergoing cardiac surgery are relatively elderly, with hypertension, coronary artery disease and/or other forms of structural heart disease, it is not surprising that these patients have an increased risk of AF in the perioperative period. Nevertheless, the temporal relationship of cardiac surgery with the development of the arrhythmia in patients both with and without a history of AF, clearly points to the presence of precipitants of AF during the perioperative period.

AF also complicates noncardiac surgery, though less commonly than cardiac surgery. It is instructive to consider why AF might occur with noncardiac surgery, because undoubtedly some of these pathophysiologic processes contribute to AF after cardiac surgery (Table 2). Atrial fibrillation complicates major, nonthoracic surgery

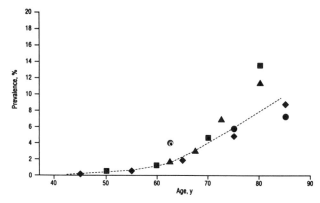

Figure 1. Estimated prevalence of atrial fibrillation at various ages (dotted line), based on data from Framingham (diamonds) [81], Cardiovascular Study Group (circles) [82], Mayo Clinic Study (squares) [83] and Busselton, Western Australia (triangles) [84]. Reproduced with permission, from Feinberg et al. [5], Arch Int Med 1995;155:469-473, copyright 1995 American Medical Association.

in approximately 5% of cases (Figure 2) [9,10]. Because cardiac and pericardial structures are not surgically manipulated, precipitating causes of AF must be indirect. Potential etiologies may include volume expansion leading to acute atrial stretch, and atrial and/or ventricular ischemia. In addition, sympathetic stimulation, in part due to perioperative pain, may alter atrial refractoriness and increase automaticity, both potentially arrhythmogenic. Metabolic and electrolyte abnormalities may also contribute to postoperative arrhythmias.

Atrial fibrillation is considerably more common after noncardiac thoracic surgery compared with major nonthoracic surgery, occurring in up to 20% of cases [11,12]. In addition to the general surgical considerations described, other conditions may exist after thoracic surgery which increase the likelihood of postoperative AF. Pericardial manipulation and irritation leading to pericarditis may occur, potentially precipitating AF. Altered pulmonary vascular capacity and resistance may increase right heart pressures and induce right atrial stretch, resulting in alteration and/or heterogeneity of atrial electrical properties. Patients with acquired lung pathology, especially smoking related disorders, may be at increased risk for chronic obstructive lung disease and consequent pulmonary hypertension, as well as coexisting coronary artery disease (CAD), all of which may increase the risk of atrial arrhythmias.

Following cardiac surgery, the incidence of AF is higher. These patients share risks as described above for other operations, and acquire new risks unique to cardiac surgery. While reports vary regarding the overall incidence of AF due to differences in patient selection, definitions of AF duration, and surveillance techniques, coronary artery bypass grafting (CABG) is complicated by AF in approximately 30% of cases [3,4,13]. Among patients with a preoperative history of AF, the postoperative AF risk increases two-fold [3]. Further increases in postoperative AF accompany aortic and mitral valve operations, especially when

Table 1. Odds Ratios for Developing Atrial Fibrillation

Risk Factor	Men (n=2090)	Women (n=1641)
Age (per decade)	2.1	2.2
Congestive heart failure	4.5	5.9
Valvular heart disease	1.8	3.4
Hypertension	1.5	1.4
Diabetes	1.4	1.6
Myocardial infarction	1.4	Ns

Odds ratios for disorders related to the development of atrial fibrillation within the Framingham population, $p<0.05$, unless noted. Abbreviation: ns= non-significant. Adapted with permission from Benjamin et al. [6], JAMA 1994;271:840-844, copyright 1994, American Medical Association.

combined with CABG or operation on more than one valve [3,13].

That the risk of AF after cardiac surgery exceeds that of thoracic surgery in part be due to the associated extensive pericardiotomy, venous cannulation [4], and cardiopulmonary bypass. Cardiopulmonary bypass may contribute to pathophysiological changes including electrolyte and metabolic abnormalities, incomplete atrial cardioplegic protection, and reperfusion injury. Hypomagnesemia may be present during and following cardiopulmonary bypass [14,15,16], and may promote AF largely through influences on potassium and calcium homeostasis. In addition, achieving complete atrial cardioplegic protection has proven difficult [17,18]; atrial mechanical activity has been demonstrated during cardioplegic arrest [19,20]. Inadequate protection from ischemia may increase AF risk by altering atrial electrical and mechanical function. Ischemia-reperfusion injury may accompany cardiopulmonary bypass [21]. Triiodothyronine (T3) supplementation may attenuate this process, reducing the incidence of postoperative AF [22]. The clinical relevance of ischemia-reperfusion injury in general remains controversial, and agents such as nitric oxide and adenosine that may be capable of attenuating ischemia-reperfusion injury have not been studied in relation to postoperative AF.

New postoperative AF occurred in nearly one half of the patients undergoing aortic valve replacement in Creswell's series [3]. However, preoperative AF was more than 5 times as common in patients undergoing aortic valve surgery compared to CABG [3]. Thus, aortic valve disease heightens vulnerability to AF in both the pre- and perioperative periods. The increased risk may stem from atrial and ventricular hypertrophy, chronic diastolic abnormalities of the left ventricle leading to reduced ventricular compliance, myocardial ischemia and/or elevated left atrial pressure. Intraoperatively, ventricular hypertrophy may hinder adequate left ventricular myocardial preservation, potentiating ischemia and diastolic abnormalities causing further elevation of left atrial pressures. Finally, as with CABG, age is a powerful predictor of AF after aortic valve surgery [3,23].

Of all cardiac surgical procedures, mitral valve surgery carries the greatest hazard of postoperative AF [3,13]. Of course, mitral stenosis and regurgitation frequently lead to AF before surgery. Acute and chronic mitral valve disorders may induce atrial dilatation and increase pulmonary capillary and left atrial pressures, which can contribute to the development of AF. In addition, with rheumatic mitral disease, atrial myopathic processes may occur, producing a substrate of electrical heterogenity, and hence AF. Thus, preoperative changes in the left atrium due to the hemodynamic effects of the mitral pathology factor importantly in the vulnerability of these patients to develop AF, both prior to and after cardiac surgery. In addition, the operative approach to the mitral valve itself traumatizes the atria and likely contributes to the risk of AF. Atriotomy may affect atrial electrical properties, and could disrupt atrial arterial supply, including the sinus node artery. Of interest, postoperative AF appears to occur as commonly with mitral valve repair as with mitral valve replacement [3,13]. Various atriotomy approaches to mitral valve exposure appear to have similar incidences of postoperative AF [24,25].

Not all cardiac surgical procedures are complicated by high rates of AF, however. AF complicates surgical repair of congenital heart anomalies less frequently than CABG or valvular surgery. Atrial septal defect closure, for example, is complicated by AF in approximately 15% of cases [3]. Following the Fontan procedure, the prevalence is somewhat higher [26,27]. These overall lower incidences of AF occur despite extensive atrial surgery, and may relate to a more normal atrial ultrastructure. The younger age, lower prevalence of concomitant coronary disease, and less atrial fibrosis and/or dilatation all probably protect against postoperative AF in these patients. That AF appears to be less common in small hearts has been substantiated in veterinary studies [28], and presumably relates to a critical amount of atrial myocardium large enough to support the multiple simultaneous reentry circuits necessary to maintain AF. Thus, the smaller atrial size common in pediatric surgery likely confers some resistance to postoperative AF. This concept is used in the Maze procedure, which compartmentalizes the atria, thereby reducing the expanse of contiguous atrial tissue so that multiple reentry circuits cannot occur simultaneously, precluding AF [29].

Atrial fibrillation also occurs relatively infrequently following cardiac transplantation, on the order of 11% [3]. Donor hearts generally originate from younger persons and screening procedures assure significant cardiovascular disease is absent. Thus, despite extensive atrial surgery, pericardiotomy, and cardiopulmonary bypass, there is relatively little AF, attesting to the importance of the underling atrial substrate in the development of the arrhythmia.

Newer approaches to cardiac surgery may affect the prevalence of postoperative AF. The absence of cardiopulmonary bypass may limit the risk of postoperative AF following minimally invasive CABG. Preliminary data from minimally invasive CABG suggest perioperative AF incidence of 0 to 8.0 % [30,31,32]. Other potential explanations for reduced AF after minimally invasive CABG include less pericardial manipulation and less postoperative pain. To this point, however, minimally invasive approaches to valve surgery have not impacted on the incidence of postoperative AF. In summary, for patients undergoing cardiac surgery, it seems likely the underlying cardiac pathology plays a prominent role in establishing the vulnerability to AF, and certain precipitants encountered during and following the operation act to induce the arrhythmia. After a brief review of the general pathophysiology of AF, this chapter will review in greater depth several acquired anatomic and electrophysiologic abnormalities of the atria, in particular aging and ischemia. This chapter will also review potential precipitants for AF in cardiac surgical patients, such as altered autonomic balance, atrial ischemia, electrolyte abnormalities, and pericarditis.

2. Anatomic and Physiologic Basis of a Trial Fibrillation

Atrial fibrillation requires both an initiating factor(s) and a substrate capable of maintaining the arrhythmia. Although AF can frequently be induced with premature atrial stimulation in the electrophysiology laboratory, it is typically nonsustained in patients without prior clinical history of AF. Thus, both triggering and substrate issues must be considered.

Atrial fibrillation occurs as a result of multiple re-entry circuit wavelets in the atria [33]. Approximately 4 to 6 simultaneous reentrant wavelets are necessary to maintain AF [34]. These wavelets are propagated around areas of functional or anatomical conduction block or delay. The wavelets' electrophysiological properties

Table 2. Potential Pathologic Factors for Developing Postoperative Atrial Fibrillation

Patient Groups

Pathologic Factor	Preoperative/ Nonoperative	Nonthoracic Surgery	Thoracic Surgery	CABG	Valve Surgery
Cardiac Factors					
Age-Related Atrial Abnormalities	+	+	+	+	+
Mitral or Tricuspid Valve Disorders	+	+	+	+	+
Aortic Valve Disorders	+	+	+	+	+
Systemic Hypertension	+	+	+	+	+
Pulmonary Hypertension	+	+	+	+	+
Cardiomyopathy, Dilated or Infiltrative	+	+	+	+	+
Chronic CAD or Prior MI	+	+	+	+	+
Pericarditis	+	+	+	+	+
Non Cardiac Factors					
Sympathetic Stimulation	+	+	+	+	+
Chronic Obstructive Lung Disease	+	+	+	+	+
Parasympathetic Stimulation	+	+	(+)	(+)	(+)
Hyperthyroidism	+	+	+	+	+
Idiopathic	+	+	+	+	+
Perioperative Factors					
Acute Atrial Stretch due to Volume Expansion		+	+	+	+
Catecholamine Excess		+	+	+	+
β- Blocker Withdrawal		+	+	+	+
Postoperative MI or Ischemia		+	+	+	+
Electrolyte or Metabolic Derangements		+	+	+	+
Pericardial Manipulation/ Irritation			+	+	+
Hypoxia			+	+	+
Increased Pulmonary Vascular Resistance			+	+	+
Cardiopulmonary Bypass				+	+
Atrial Ischemia				+	+
Atriotomy and Cannulation				+	+
Pericardiotomy/ Pericarditis				+	+
Preexisting Atrial and/or Ventricular changes due to Effects of Valve Disorder					+
Extensive Atrial Surgery					+

Abbreviations: CABG, coronary artery bypass grafting; CAD, coronary artery disease; MI, myocardial infarction. Symbols: +, potential factor; (+), of theoretical importance, but observational support lacking

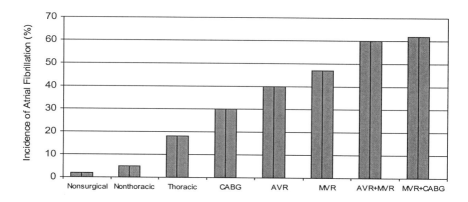

Figure 2. Incidence of Atrial Fibrillation in Surgical Populations. Abbreviations: CABG, coronary artery bypass grafting; AVR, aortic valve replacement; MVR, mitral valve repair/replacement

are defined by conduction velocity and refractory period. Slow conduction allows proximal parts of circuits to recover; short refractory periods permit rapid recovery of excitability. Thus, processes that slow conduction velocity or shorten the refractory period facilitate AF. The wavelets must be of sufficient size to permit recovery of excitability ahead of the wavefront. The likelihood of developing sustained AF increases with larger atrial size at least in part due to a larger area available to the simultaneous wavelets [8]. Conversely, small atria may not support multiple simultaneous wavelets, and thus resist AF. In response to pathophysiologic influences, such as hypertension, CAD and cardiomyopathy, fibrous and fatty tissues are deposited in the atria [35]. To some degree, this also occurs with normal aging, as well. These changes are frequently patchy, and result in areas of slowed or blocked conduction, nonhomogenous anisotropy, and dispersion of atrial refractoriness, producing a substrate conducive to reentry.

Atrial flutter, in contrast to the multiple reentry circuits of AF, typically utilizes a single macroreentry circuit in the right atrium. Atrial flutter occurs relatively commonly after cardiac surgery; atrial tachycardia is less common. Both occur less frequently than AF. Most studies after cardiac surgery do not differentiate among these arrhythmias. Potential etiologies of AF are believed to be generally applicable to each, though the electrophysiologic mechanisms differ.

Anatomically, the atrial myocardium differs significantly from the ventricular myocardium. First, several anatomic obstacles - superior and inferior venea cavae, coronary sinus ostium, pulmonary venous ostia, eustacian ridge - interrupt the atrial myocardium, necessitating paths around these for synchronous atrial electrical activation. Secondly, the atria contain both smooth and trabeculated tissue, each with differing conduction properties. At a cellular level, end to end conduction is more rapid than side to side conduction, even in normal tissue. As a result, normal atrial conduction preferentially follows well-developed muscle bundles, such as the crista terminalis and interatrial band (Bachmann's Bundle) [36]. Thirdly, with aging, nonuniform replacement of atrial tissue with hypertrophic, sclerotic, and fatty tissues alters atrial electrophysiologic properties [35].

Pathologic processes may alter these normal anatomical and physiological atrial relationships. For example, congestive heart failure is associated with increased atrial thinning that may increase anisotropy, enhancing the vulnerability to AF [37]. It is conceivable that all or virtually all patients that develop AF in the postoperative setting have underlying atrial abnormalities. In this regard, atrial histopathological changes were recently reported in 12 of 12 patients with idiopathic AF, despite absence of evidence of heart disease on routine diagnostic studies [8]. Further, during right atrial programmed stimulation in the preoperative period, AF may be induced, suggesting a preexisting substrate conducive to AF [38]. Patients with inducible AF have a high risk of AF after cardiac surgery. Moreover, the inability to induce AF strongly predicts freedom from postoperative AF [38].

In nonoperative patients, left atrial enlargement is associated with a higher incidence of AF [7]. Beyond the atrial size alone, however, the process responsible for atrial enlargement may be a more important predictor of risk for AF. With regard to AF after cardiac surgery, the importance of left atrial enlargement is less clear. In Mathew et al. series [4], preoperative echocardiographic assessment of left atrial size did not predict AF after CABG. However, few data exist regarding whether the etiology or severity of atrial dilatation enhances AF vulnerability after cardiac surgery.

Acute perioperative atrial enlargement might increase postoperative AF risk. Patients undergoing cardiac, or any major surgical procedures, may be subjected to rapidly changing hemodynamic stresses such as volume loading, with subsequent acute atrial stretch. Volume loading produces acute atrial stretch and facilitates AF [39]. Importantly, atrial stretch occurs heterogeneously, stretching thin areas more than thick areas. At baseline, the effective refractory period in the thick crista terminalis exceeds that of the thin free right atrial wall. With volume loading and differential stretch, however, this difference in effective refractory periods is accentuated. During this period of increased dispersion of refractoriness, AF is more easily induced [39]. These findings may explain the observation that modest increases in mean central venous pressure are associated with increases in risk of postoperative AF [40]. While this data would reflect right atrial stretch, similar mechanisms may apply to the left atrium as well.

The electrocardiographic P wave reflects atrial conduction and size. Because atrial conduction abnormalities predispose to AF, P wave duration identifies patients at risk for AF. Buxton and Josephson [41] measured total P wave duration from electrocardiograph leads I, II and III, and reported an association with postoperative AF. Similarly, abnormal long signal-averaged P wave electrocardiograms predict postoperative AF [42,43]. While the predictive value of P wave analysis by either means is at best moderate, these findings underscore the importance of underlying atrial conduction abnormalities in the genesis of postoperative AF.

3. Specific Clinical Pathophysiologic Factors

3.1. Age

Advanced age is the most consistent predictor of developing AF after cardiac surgery [3,4,13,44]. Aging is also related to the development of AF in the non-surgical population [5]. These data are illustrated in figure 1.

Aging is accompanied by structural and electrical changes in the atria that may provide a substrate conducive to AF. Changes begin in infancy, with endocardial hypertrophy characterized by focal or diffuse areas of smooth muscle cell, elastic and/or collagen proliferation [35]. During adult life, progressive sclerotic changes develop within the atrial endocardium, myocardium, and epicardium resulting in fragmentation, dissolution of distinct endocardial layers, infiltration of elastic and collagenous elements, and atrophy of atrial myocytes [35]. Many of these changes are heterogenous with respect to both location and timing. These structural changes promote intraatrial conduction delay, conduction block, nonuniform anisotropy and dispersion of refractoriness.

Age related conduction and repolarization abnormalities have been demonstrated in tissue excised from the right atrium during aortic valve replacement [23]. Tissue samples from patients 20 years and younger demonstrated normal atrial transmembrane potentials and synchronous contraction without conduction abnormalities. In contrast, samples from patients 40 years or older exhibited a reduction in resting membrane potential, decrease in total action potential amplitude and duration, slower maximal velocity of conduction, and more rapid repolarization. Tissue from older patients exhibited spontaneous phase 4 depolarizations which were absent in the younger group. In addition, Spach and Dobler [45] noted age-dependent electrical uncoupling of side-to-side atrial connections. Older patients exhibited an increase in the longitudinal conduction velocity and a decrease in transverse velocity compared to younger patients. As a consequence, previously uniform anisotropic conduction was replaced in older patients with nonuniform anisotropic conduction. Aging may also result in an increased dispersion of atrial refractoriness [46]. The changes in atrial refractoriness may result from altered autonomic innervation or primary changes within the atrial myocytes [46].

Finally, age related ventricular changes may affect AF vulnerability. Reduced ventricular compliance can increase atrial volumes and pressures. These influences may be particularly relevant in light of perioperative changes in ventricular loading conditions. Atrial stretch may be an important cause of new onset AF [39].

Thus, advancing age, a strong predictor of postoperative AF, provides a substrate conducive to the arrhythmia. This substrate is characterized by patchy fibrosis causing slow conduction, nonuniform anisotropy and increased dispersion of atrial refractoriness.

3.2. Atrial ischemia

Atrial ischemia may contribute to the development of AF after cardiac surgery in two ways. First, chronic atrial ischemia or infarction can produce structural changes in the atrium. For example, chronic CAD may intensify sclerotic changes. Secondly, acute atrial ischemia may induce electrophysiologic and/or mechanical abnormalities that might favor the development of AF.

Electrophysiologically, acute ischemia slows and fractionates conduction by depolarizing membranes, slowing action potential upstroke, and decreasing action potential duration [45]. The refractory periods initially shorten, then lengthen, and dispersion of refractoriness increases [47]. Such electrophysiologic changes could favor the development of AF. However, atrial ischemic injury is difficult to demonstrate clinically. Acute atrial ischemia could develop with cardiac surgery from inadequate cardioplegic protection [18,48] or compromised atrial coronary arterial supply [49,50].

Some investigators have hypothesized that much of postoperative AF is attributable to inadequate atrial protection during cold potassium cardioplegia [48]. Smith et al. [18] measured atrial temperatures during antegrade cold potassium cardioplegic arrest. Atrial temperatures substantially exceeded ventricular temperatures, possibly related to the circulation of systemic blood through the atria during bypass and the superficial location of the atria within the operative field. Atrial mechanical activity can be demonstrated during cold cardioplegic arrest [19,20], implying incomplete electromechanical arrest. Atrial ischemia may develop, therefore, due to persistent metabolic activity during bypass.

In an attempt to determine if higher atrial temperatures lead to postoperative supraventricular arrhythmias, Yousif et al. [51] augmented atrial cooling by applying topical cold slush to 12 randomly selected patients from 100 patients undergoing CABG. Seven (58%) of the 12 patients developed postoperative atrial arrhythmias, compared to only 19% of the control patients who did not have augmented atrial cooling. Other data suggest augmentation of atrial hypothermia with topical cooling does not reduce the incidence of AF when compared to intermittent aortic cross clamping [52]. However, atrial temperatures were not recorded in either study, and it is conceivable that either excessive cooling may have caused atrial injury, or that inadequate cooling failed to prevent atrial injury. Indeed, Smith et al. [18] demonstrated only brief reductions in atrial septal temperature with intermittent topical cooling. No form of cardioplegia appears to protect the heart completely, or provide particular protection from postoperative AF. Using biochemical markers, Yau et al. [17] demonstrated incomplete ischemic protection with multiple commonly used cardioplegic methods. Thus, it remains uncertain what role, if any, inadequate hypothermic protection has in the genesis of postoperative AF.

In nonoperative patients, right coronary artery stenosis have been suggested to relate to the development of AF [53,54]. Supraventricular arrhythmias, particularly AF, accompany atrial infarction [53] and right ventricular ischemic injury [54]. An association between right coronary artery disease and AF has also been reported in patients following CABG in some [49,50] but not all series [4].

3.3. Autonomic nervous system

Autonomic influences affect atrial vulnerability to AF. However, the interactions and balance of vagal and sympathetic influences postoperatively are complex and difficult to study. Vagal stimulation causes uneven shortening of atrial refractoriness, and may contribute to increased dispersion of refractoriness with a subsequent vulnerability to AF [55]. Some paroxysms of AF in the nonoperative setting may be triggered by hypervagotonia [46]. Thoracic surgery could lead to vagal irritation and hyperactivity, though bradycardia reflective of excessive vagal tone is seldom seen prior to the onset of AF after cardiac surgery. In fact, vagal withdrawal as measured by heart rate variability may precede AF after CABG [56].

Alternatively, paroxysms of AF may be sympathetically triggered [46]. Indeed, β– adrenergic stimulation both increases atrial ectopy, which may trigger AF, and shortens atrial refractoriness, providing a more conducive substrate for AF. In contrast to vagally mediated AF, however, sympathetically driven AF is more common in structurally abnormal hearts and tends to be preceded by physical or emotional stresses and an increase in heart rate [46]. Intraoperatively, endogenous catecholamine levels peak at time of cross-clamp removal [57]. Postoperative sympathetic activity may be further increased from exogenous catecholamines administered to support blood pressure and contractility. After cardiac surgery, additional endogenous catecholamine release may occur in response to pain and emotional stress, or in support of inadequate hemodynamics. An additional source of cardiac adrenergic stimulation originates from the sympathetic ganglia, which may exert nonhomogenous cardiac effects.

Clinical observations certainly support an association between sympathetic activity and the development of AF after cardiac surgery, though isolating the proarrhythmic effects of the increased sympathetic tone from the patient's condition that produced the increased sympathetic tone is difficult. In patients experiencing AF after cardiac surgery, norepinephrine levels are elevated compared to patients who do not develop AF [58]. Moreover, pre- or post-cardiopulmonary bypass use of exogenous inotropic agents increases AF risk [4]. Premature atrial beats, the proximate trigger for AF, are increased with elevated sympathetic tone [58]. Frost et al [59] also noted an increase in heart rate and atrial ectopy preceding the development of AF in the postoperative period. Heart rate variability findings suggesting sympathetic activation precede AF after CABG [56].

Additional evidence supporting a role of sympathetic stimulation comes from trials aimed at postoperative AF prevention with β-blockers. Beta-blockers suppress automaticity, prolong refractory periods, and slow conduction velocity. These effects may protect against AF. While many data suggest that β-blockade protects against AF after cardiac surgery [60] and noncardiac thoracic surgery [61], a stronger case exists that β-blocker withdrawal increases AF risk. This may result from a hypersensitivity to catecholamines due to cellular adaptations to chronic β- blocker exposure. Kempf et al. [62] demonstrated an increase in β-adrenergic receptor density in excised atrial tissue from patients treated with β-blockers. The increased receptor density may amplify the effects of catecholamine stimulation in the absence of receptor blockade postoperatively, and increased sensitivity to catecholamines is observed in patients withdrawn from β-blocking agents [63]. Further, enhanced sensitivity to catecholamines can be demonstrated with inhibition of endothelial derived nitric oxide [55], though the association between nitric oxide metabolism with cardiopulmonary bypass and AF after cardiac surgery has not been studied.

3.4. Electrolyte abnormalities

Perioperative derangements in potassium and magnesium homeostasis may contribute to postoperative arrhythmias [15,16]. Magnesium has received considerable attention regarding its potential roles in the genesis of postoperative AF, and for magnesium supplementation to protect against arrhythmia. Several studies have documented hypomagnesemia following cardiopulmonary bypass [14,15,16,64]. Some clinical trials suggest that administration of magnesium salts may lessen the frequency of perioperative atrial and ventricular dysrhythmias [16,16,64], although other studies have failed to demonstrate such a benefit [65].

Despite the submillimolar activity of myocardial intracellular magnesium, changes in its concentration can have major effects on potassium and calcium movement through magnesium dependent ion channels. These processes have been summarized previously [15,66]. In brief, the transmembrane potassium gradient is maintained through a magnesium dependent membrane sodium- potassium ATPase. A reduction in intracellular magnesium limits the ability of this channel and other potassium channels to maintain inward rectification of potassium. Indeed, significant myocellular potassium loss is usually accompanied by magnesium depletion, and correction of the hypokalemia usually requires concurrent magnesium replacement.

In addition, magnesium regulates the slow transsarcolemmal calcium inflow proceeding via L-type calcium channels and sarcoplasmic reticulum calcium handling. A decrease in intracellular magnesium enhances inward calcium flux [66]. Abnormalities in intracellular calcium may effect contractile and electrophysiologic properties.

Risk factors for hypomagnesemia include congestive heart failure, diabetes mellitus and loop diuretic use [67]; many patients with these features undergo cardiac surgery. Hypomagnesemia occurs during cardiopulmonary bypass and the first postoperative day, and tends to normalize in patients between postoperative days 2 and 4 [15,16]. Magnesium loss after cardiac surgery may occur from dilutional effects and/or increased magnesium excretion [68].

Unfortunately, studies of magnesium are complicated by difficulties in assaying ionized magnesium, the biologically important species. Serum magnesium levels have correlated poorly with tissue magnesium levels from the right atrial appendage [69] or serum ultrafilterable magnesium [14].

In summary, it remains possible that hypomagnesemia, a condition common in patients undergoing CABG and likely exacerbated by cardiopulmonary bypass, plays a role in the pathogenesis of AF after cardiac surgery, and that supplementation may confer some degree of protection.

3.5. Pericarditis

A model of sterile pericarditis producing AF or flutter has been developed [70]. Pericarditis may cause atrial epicardial inflammatory injury and a substrate for AF [71]. Spodick [72] studied 100 consecutive clinical cases of pericarditis of various etiologies, though, and found AF in only 7 patients, each of whom had underlying heart disease. These findings may cast doubt on the direct role of pericarditis in causing AF. Alternatively, underlying atrial pathology may create a substrate vulnerable to AF when exposed to pericarditis. Thus, it is possible that patients undergoing cardiac surgery have atrial abnormalities that serve to increase vulnerability to AF when challenged by pericarditis, similar to those described by Spodick. In addition, the risk of AF after non-cardiac thoracic surgery appears to be increased when the pericardium is manipulated surgically [11].

Additional evidence supporting a role for pericarditis derives from the implantable cardioverter-defibrillator (ICD) literature. Epicardial ICD implantation resulted in significantly more postoperative AF (9%) than transvenous ICD implantation (<1%), and pericardial irritation may be responsible for the increased risk [73]. That epicardial implantation requires sternotomy or thoracotomy also must be considered, though, as thoracotomy itself appears to carry a risk of AF similar to that of epicardial ICD implantation [11].

Although pericarditis is assumed to be common following cardiac surgery because of the inherent pericardiotomy, few studies have examined its relationship to postoperative AF. In 123 patients after CABG, pericarditis, defined as the presence of a pericardial friction rub heard by two observers on two occasions, was present in 41% of the patients [74]. However, pericarditis was not predictive of the development of AF. Crosby et al. [75] found clinical pericarditis in only 7% of patients following CABG and also detected no association between pericarditis and postoperative AF. Similarly, pericardial effusions after cardiac surgery have been suggested to be associated with the development of AF [76]. Studies demonstrating more complete pericardial drainage, however, yielded conflicting data on the incidence of postoperative atrial arrhythmias [76,77,78].

Conceivably, more intense pericardial inflammation may be associated with larger effusions and a higher incidence of postoperative AF, though this remains speculative. Firm conclusions about the role of pericarditis in postoperative AF cannot be made from the available data.

4. Timing of Atrial Fibrillation After Cardiac Surgery

One aspect of the pathogenesis of AF after cardiac surgery that is particularly poorly understood involves the timing of AF onset. Multiple studies indicate the development of postoperative AF peaks between the second and third postoperative day. Understanding this phenomena might yield a more thorough understanding of the pathogenesis of postoperative AF. Thus far, no convincing explanation has been forwarded. In fact, given the mechanisms felt to be responsible for triggering postoperative AF, one would expect the arrhythmia to characteristically occur earlier in the postoperative period.

In β-adrenergic blocker withdrawn patients, the pharmacological activity of the agent may be sufficiently low about this time to increase the sensitivity to catecholamines, and thus increase the vulnerability to develop AF. While this may be true, postoperative AF appears to follow a similar time frame in patients who are continued on β- blockers postoperatively, as well as in patients that do not receive β-blockers at all. Sympathetic activity appears to fall after peaking during cardiopulmonary bypass [57], though may increase again just prior to AF onset [56,59].

Magnesium homeostasis is usually abnormal between the second and third postoperative day, though the serum measured magnesium is not as low as intraoperatively, or earlier in the postoperative course [15,16]. If disordered magnesium homeostasis were causative, one might expect the earlier, more severe disturbances to translate into an earlier peak incidence of AF.

Volume expansion and volume shifts occur over the first several postoperative days. Yet once again, volume expansion is likely to be most severe in the early postoperative period, and therefore it may be difficult to implicate this factor for the observed timing.

The time response of atrial myocardium to ischemia is less well characterized than ventricular myocardium. However, when AF complicates acute myocardial infarction, its occurrence is usually early, typically within first 3 to 12 hours [79,80]. Atrial fibrillation occurring greater than 24 hours after infarction tends to reflect secondary elevations in left atrial pressure resulting from left ventricular dysfunction or mitral regurgitation, rather than ongoing ischemia [81]. These observations would tend to argue against delayed ischemia and/or arrhythmic response to ischemic injury. Any potential role of ischemia-reperfusion injury or recovery from cardiopulmonary bypass remains entirely speculative.

Finally, if pericarditis is an important contributor to postoperative AF, it may take time to develop a maximal inflammatory response. The timing of pericarditis after cardiac surgery has not been well characterized, however.

5. Conclusion

Although AF after cardiac surgery is an extremely common problem, its pathogenesis and timing are incompletely understood. In most, if not all cases, underlying structural and/or electrical abnormalities of the atria are present preoperatively. These abnormalities are commonly related to aging as well as the accompanying cardiac disease, resulting in electrophysiologic abnormalities including more nonhomogeneous anisotropy, shortening of refractoriness, and dispersion of refractoriness. In general, the preoperative degree of underlying structural and electrical abnormalities either clinically overt or subtle, probably correlates with the propensity to develop postoperative AF. In the perioperative period, the vulnerability to AF is modified by factors such as atrial ischemia, acute atrial stretch, electrolyte imbalances, heightened sympathetic tone and pericarditis, producing an electrophysiologic milieu suitable to the maintenance of AF following atrial ectopic triggers.

References

1. Prystowsky EN, Benson DW, Fuster V, et al. Management of patients with atrial fibrillation. Circulation 1996;93:1262-1277.
2. Cameron A, Schwartz ML, Kronmal RA, Kosinski AS. Prevalence and significance of atrial fibrillation in coronary artery disease (CASS registry). Am J Cardiol 1988;61:714-717.
3. Creswell LL, Schuessler RB, Rosenbloom M, Cox JL. Hazards of postoperative atrial arrhythmias. Ann Thorac Surg 1993:56;539-545.
4. Mathew JP, Parks R, Savino JS, et al. Atrial fibrillation following coronary artery bypass graft surgery. JAMA 1996;274:300-306.
5. Feinberg WM, Blackshear JL, Laupacis A, Kronmal R, Hart RG. Prevalence, age distribution, and gender of patients with atrial fibrillation; analysis and implications. Arch Int Med 1995;155:469-473.
6. Benjamin EJ, Levy D, Vaziri SM, D'Agostino RB, Belanger AJ, Wolf PA. Independent risk factors for atrial fibrillation in a population-based cohort. JAMA 1994;271:840-844.
7. Psaty BM, Manolio TA, Kuller LH, et al. Incidence of and risk factors for atrial fibrillation in older adults. Circulation 1997;96:2455-2461.
8. Frustaci A, Chimenti C, Bellocci F, Morgante E, Russo MA, Maseri A. Histological substrate of atrial biopsies in patients with lone atrial fibrillation. Circulation 1997;96:1180-1184.
9. Johnston KW. Multicenter prospective study of non ruptured abdominal aortic aneurysm, part II; Variables predicting morbidity and mortality. J Vasc Surg 1989;9:437-447.
10. Goldman L. Supraventricular tachyarrythmias in hospitalized adults after surgery. Clinical correlates in patients over 40 years of age after major noncardiac surgery. Chest 1978;73:450-454.
11. Beck-Nielsen J, Sorensen HR, Alstrip P. Atrial fibrillation following thoracotomy for non-cardiac diseases, in particular lung cancer. Acta Med Scand 1973;193:425-429.
12. von Knorring J, Lepantalo M, Lindgren L, Lindfors O. Cardiac arrhythmias and myocardial ischemia after thoracotomy for lung cancer. Ann Thorac Surg 1992;53:642-647.
13. Almassi GH, Schowalter T, Nicolosi AC, et al. Atrial fibrillation after cardiac surgery; a major morbid event? Ann Surg 1997;226:501-515.
14. Aglio LS, Stanford GG, Maddi R, Boyd III JL, Nussbaum S, Chernow B. Hypomagnesemia is common following cardiac surgery. J Cardiothorac Vasc Anesth 1991;5:201-208.
15. Casthely PA, Yoganathan T, Komer C, Kelly M. Magnesium and arrhythmias after coronary artery bypass surgery. J Cardiothorac Vasc Anesth 1994;8:188-191.
16. Fanning WJ, Thomas CS, Roach A, Tomichek R, Alford WC, Stoney WS. Prophylaxis of atrial fibrillation with magnesium sulfate after coronary artery bypass grafting. Ann Thorac Surg 1991;52:529-533.
17. Yau TM, Ikonomidis JS, Weisel RD, et al. Which techniques of cardioplegia prevent ischemia? Ann Thorac Surg 1993;56:1020-1028.
18. Smith PK, Buhrman WC, Levett JM, Ferguson TB, Holman WL, Cox JL. Supraventricular conduction abnormalities following cardiac operations: a complication of inadequate atrial preservation. J Thorac Cardiovasc Surg 1983;85:105-115.
19. Tchervenkov CI, Wynands JE, Symes JS, Malcolm ID, Dobell ARC, Morin JE. Persistent atrial activity during cardioplegic arrest: a possible factor in the etiology of postoperative supraventricular tachyarrhythmias. Ann Thorac Surg 1983;36:437-443.
20. Mullen JC, Khan N, Weisel RD, et al. Atrial activity during cardioplegia and postoperative arrhythmias. J Thorac Cardiovasc Surg 1987;94:558-565.
21. Hansen PR. Myocardial reperfusion injury: experimental evidence and clinical relevance. Eur H Jour. 1995;16:734-740.
22. Klemperer JD, Klein IL, Ojamaa K, et al. Triiodothronine therapy lowers the incidence of atrial fibrillation after cardiac operations. Ann Thor Surg 1996;61:1323-1329.

23. Bush HL, Gelband H. Hoffman BF, Malm JR. Electrophysiological basis for supraventricular arrhythmias following surgical procedures for aortic stenosis. Arch Surg 1971;103:620-625.
24. Masuda M, Tominaga R, Kawachi Y, et al. Postoperative cardiac rhythms with superior-septal approach and lateral approach to the mitral valve. Ann Thorac Surg 1996;62:1118-1122.
25. Tambeur L, Meyns B, Flameng W, Daenen W. Rhythm disturbances after mitral valve surgery: comparison between left atrial and extended trans-septal approach. Cardiovasc Surg 1996:6;820-824.
26. Peters NS, Somerville J. Arrhythmias after the Fontan procedure. Br Heart J. 1992;68-199-204.
27. Balaji S, Gewillig M, Bull C, de Leval M, Deanfield JE. Arrhythmias after the Fontan procedure. Comparison of the total cavopulmonary connection and atriopulmonary connection. Circulation 1996;84[suppl III]:III-162-III-167.
28. Buchanan JW. Spontaneous arrhythmia and conduction disturbances in domestic animals. Ann NY Acad Sci 1965;127:224-238.
29. Cox JL, Boineau JP, Schuessler RB, Jaquiss RDB, Lappas DG. Modification of the maze procedure for atrial flutter and atrial fibrillation: I. Rationale and surgical results. J Thorac Cardiovasc Surg 1995;110:473-484.
30. Allen KB, Matheny RG, Robison RJ, Heimansohn DA, Shaar CJ. Minimally invasive versus conventional reoperative coronary artery bypass. Ann Thorac Surg 1997;64:616-622.
31. Calafiore AM, Di Giammarco G, Teodori G, et al. Midterm results after minimally invasive coronary surgery (LAST operation). J Thorac Cardiovasc Surg 1998;115:763-770.
32. Stanbridge RD, Hadjinikolaou LK, Cohen AS, Foale RA, Davies WD, Kutoubi AA. Minimally invasive coronary revascularization through parasternal incisions without cardiopulmonary bypass. Ann Thorac Surg 1997;63 (Suppl 6);S53-S56.
33. Moe GK. On the multiple wavelet hypothesis of atrial fibrillation. Arch Int Pharmacodyn Ther 1962;140:183-188.
34. Allessie MA. Reentrant mechanisms undelying atrial fibrillation. In: Zipes DP, Jalife J, eds. Cardiac Electrophysiology: from cell to bedside. WB Saunders, Philadelphia, 1995, p. 562-566.
35. Bharati S and Lev M. Histology of the normal and diseased atrium. In: Falk RH, Podrid PJ, eds. Atrial Fibrillation; mechanisms and management. Raven Press, New York, 1992, p. 15-39.
36. Janse MJ and Allessie MA. Experimental observations in atrial fibrillation. In: Falk RH and Podrid PJ, eds. Atrial Fibrillation; mechanisms and management. Raven Press, New York, 1992, p. 41-57.
37. Schussler RB, Boineau JP, Bromberg BI, Hand DE, Yamauchi S, Cox, JL. In: Zipes DP, Jaliff J, eds. Cardiac Electrophysiology: from cell to bedside. WB Saunders, Philadelphia, 1995, p.543-561.
38. Lowe JE, Hendry PJ, Hendrickson SC, Wells R. Intraoperative identification of cardiac patients at risk to develop postoperative atrial fibrillation. Ann Surg 1991;213:388-391.
39. Satoh T, Zipes DP. Unequal atrial stretch in dogs increases dispersion of refractoriness conducive to developing atrial fibrillation. J Cardiovasc Electrophysiol 1996;7:833-842.
40. Frost L, Jacobsen CJ, Christiansen EH, et al. Hemodynamic predictors of atrial fibrillation and flutter after coronary artery bypass grafting. Acta Anaesth Scand 1995;39:690-697.
41. Buxton AE, Josephson ME. The role of the P wave duration as a predictor of postoperative atrial arrhythmia. Chest 1981;80:68-73.
42. Steinberg JS, Zelenkofske S, Wong SC, Gelernt M, Sciacca R, Menchavez E. Value of the P-wave signal-averaged ECG for predicting atrial fibrillation after cardiac surgery. Circulation 1993;88:2618-2622.
43. Klein M, Evans SJL, Blumberg S, Cataldo L, Bodenheimer MM. Use of P-wave-triggered, P-wave signal-averaged electrocardiogram to predict atrial fibrillation after coronary artery bypass surgery. Am Heart J 1995;129:895-901.
44. Fuller JA, Adams GC, Buxton B. Atrial fibrillation after coronary artery bypass grafting; is it a disorder of the elderly? J Thorac Cardiovasc Surg 1989;97:821-825.
45. Spach MS, Dolber PC. Relating extracellular potentials and their derivatives to anisotropic propagation at the microscopic level in human cardiac muscle; evidence for electrical uncoupling of side to side fiber connections with increasing age. Circ Res 1986;58:356-371.
46. Lindsay BD, Smith JM. Electrophysiologic aspects of human atrial fibrillation. Cardiol Clinics 1996;14:483-505.
47. Damiano RJ. The electrophysiology of ischemia and cardioplegia: implications for myocardial protection. J Card Surg 1995;10:445-453.
48. Cox JL. A perspective of postoperative atrial fibrillation in cardiac operations. Ann Thorac Surg 1993;56:405-409.
49. Kolvekar S, D'Souza A, Akhatar P, Reek C, Garratt C, Spyt T. Role of atrial ischaemia in development of atrial fibrillation following coronary artery bypass surgery. Eur J Cardio-Thor Surg 1997;11:70-75.

34

50. Mendes LS, Connelly GP, McKenney PA, et al. Right coronary artery stenosis: an independent predictor of atrial fibrillation after coronary artery bypass surgery. J Am Coll Cardiol 1995;25:198-202.

51. Yousif H, Davies G, Oakley CM, Peri-operative supraventricular arrhythmias in coronary bypass surgery. Int J Cardiol 1990;26:313-318.

52. Butler J, Chong JL, Rocker GM, Pillai R, Westaby S. Atrial fibrillation after coronary artery bypass grafting: a comparison of cardioplegia versus intermittent aortic cross-clamping. Eur J Cardiothorac Surg 1993;7:23-25.

53. Lazar EJ, Goldberger J, Peled H, Sherman M, Frishman W. Atrial infarction, diagnosis and management. Am Heart J 1988;116:1058-1063.

54. Rechavia E, Strasberg B, Mager A, et al. The incidence of atrial arrhythmias during inferior wall myocardial infarction with and without right ventricular involvement. Am Heart J 1992;124:387-391.

55. Zipes DP. Atrial fibrillation: from cell to bedside. J Cardiovasc Electrophysiol 1997;8:927-938.

56. Dimmer C, Tavernier R, Gjorgov N, Van Nooten G, Clement DL, Jordaens L. Variations of autonomic tone preceding onset of atrial fibrillation after coronary artery bypass grafting. Am J Cardiol 1998;82:22-25.

57. Reves J, Karp R, Buttner E, et al. Neuronal and adrenomedullary catecholamine release in response to cardiopulmonary bypass in man. Circulation 1982;66:49-55.

58. Kalman JM, Munawar M, Howes LG, et al. Atrial fibrillation after coronary artery bypass grafting is associated with sympathetic activation. Ann Thorac Surg 1995;60:1709-1715.

59. Frost L, Molgaard H, Christiansen EH, Jacobsen CJ, Pilegaard H, Thomsen PEB. Atrial ectopic activity and atrial fibrillation/flutter after coronary artery bypass surgery; a case-base study controlling for the confounding from age, β- blocker treatment, and the time distance from operation. Int J Cardiol 1995;50:153-162.

60. Andrews TC, Reimold SC, Berlin JA, Antman EM. Prevention of supraventricular arrhythmias after coronary artery bypass surgery; a meta-analysis of randomized control trials. Circulation 1991;84[suppl III]: III-236-III-244.

61. Jakobsen CJ, Billie S, Ahlburg P, Rybro L, Hjortholm K, Andresen EB. Perioperative metoprolol reduces the frequency of atrial fibrillation after thoracotomy for lung resection. J Cardiothorac Vasc Anesth 1997;11:746-751.

62. Kempf FC, Hedberg A, Molinoff P, Josephson ME. The effects of pharmacologic therapy on atrial beta-receptor density and postoperative atrial arrhythmias. Circulation 1983;68 (Suppl III):III-57.

63. Krukemyer JJ, Boudoulas H, Binkley PF, Lima JJ. Biphasic pattern of hypersensitivity following acute propranolol withdrawal in normal subjects. Life Sciences 1989;45:1547-1551.

64. England MR, Gordon G, Salem M, Chernow B. Magnesium administration and dysrhythmias after cardiac surgery. JAMA. 1992;268:2395-2402.

65. Parikka H, Toivonen L, Pellinen T, Verkkala K, Jarvinen A, Nieminen MS. The influence of intravenous magnesium sulphate on the occurrence of atrial fibrillation after coronary artery by-pass operation. Eur Heart J 1993;14:251-258.

66. Fazekas T, Scherlag BJ, Vos M, Wellens HJJ, Lazzara R. Magnesium and the heart: antiarrhythmic therapy with magnesium. Clin Cardiol 1993;16:768-774.

67. Douban S, Brodsky MA, Whang DD, Whang R. Significance of magnesium in congestive heart failure. Am Heart J 1996;132:664-671.

68. Scheinman MM, Sullivan RW, Hyatt KH. Magnesium metabolism in patients undergoing cardiopulmonary bypass. Circulation 1986;39:(Suppl I):I-235-I-241.

69. Reinhart RA, Marx JJ, Broste SK, Haas RG. Myocardial magnesium; relation to laboratory and clinical variable in patients undergoing cardiac surgery. J Am Coll Cardiol 1991;17:651-656.

70. Page PL, Plumb VJ, Okumura K, Waldo AL. A new model of atrial flutter. J Am Coll Cardiol 1986;8:872-879.

71. James TN. Diversity of histopathologic correlates of atrial fibrillation. In: Kulbertus HE, Olsson SB, Schlepper M, eds. Atrial Fibrillation. Molndal, Sweden, A.B. Hassle, 1981, p. 13-32.

72. Spodick DH. Arrhythmias during acute pericarditis: a prospective study in 100 consecutive cases. JAMA 1976;5:39-41.

73. Ong JJC, Hsu PC, Lin L, et al. Arrhythmias after cardioverter- defibrillator implantation: comparison of epicardial and transvenous systems. Am J Cardiol 1995;75:137-140.

74. Rubin DA, Nieminski KE, Reed GE, Herman MV. Predictors, prevention and long-term prognosis of atrial fibrillation after coronary artery bypass graft operations. J Thorac Cardiovasc Surg 1987;94:331-335.

75. Crosby LH, Pifalo WB, Woll KR, Burkholder JA. Risk factors for atrial fibrillation after coronary artery bypass grafting. Am J Cardiol 1990;66:1520-1522.

76. Angelini GD, Penny WJ, El-Ghamary F, West RR, Butchart EG. The incidence and significance of early pericardial effusions after open heart surgery. Eur J Cardiothorac Surg 1987;1:165-168.

77. Mulay, Kirk AJB, Angelini GD, Wisheart JD, Hutter JA. Posterior pericardiotomy reduces the incidence of supraventricular arrhythmias following coronary artery bypass surgery. Eur J Cardiothorac Surg 1995;9:150-152.

78. Asimakopoulos G, Della Santa R, Taggart DP. Effects of posterior pericardiotomy on the incidence of atrial fibrillation and chest drainage after coronary revascularization:a prospective randomized trial. J Thorac Cardiovasc Surg 1997;11:797-799.

79. Hod H, Lew AS, Keltai M, et al. Early atrial fibrillation during evolving myocardial infarction: a consequence of impaired left atrial perfusion. Circulation 1987;75:146-150.

80. Sakata K, Kurihara H, Iwamori K, et al. Clinical and prognostic significance of atrial fibrillation in acute myocardial infarction. Am J Cardiol 1997;80:1522-1527.

81. Wolf PA, Abbott RD, Kannel WB. Atrial fibrillation as an independent risk factor for stroke; the Framingham study. Stroke 1991;22:983-988.

82. Furberg CD, Psaty BM, Manolio TA, Gardin JM, Smith VE, Rautaharju RM. Prevalence of atrial fibrillation in elderly subjects; the cardiovascular health study. Am J Cardiol 1994;74:238-241.

83. Philips SJ, Whisnant J, O'Fallon WM, Frye RL. Prevalence of cardiovascular disease and diabetes in residents of Rochester, Minnesota. Mayo Clinic Proc 1990;65:344-359.

84. Lake RR, Cullen KJ, deKlerk NH, McCall MG, Rosman DL. Atrial fibrillation in an elderly population. Aust NZ J Med 1989;19:321-326.

3 INCIDENCE, TIMING AND OUTCOME OF ATRIAL TACHYARRHYTHMIAS AFTER CARDIAC SURGERY

L. Brent Mitchell, MD,
University of Calgary, Alberta, Canada

1. Introduction

Atrial tachyarrhythmias are the most common sustained arrhythmias encountered in clinical practice [1] and are expressed as atrial fibrillation, atrial flutter, or true atrial tachycardia. The mechanism of most forms of atrial fibrillation is multiple wavelet reentry [2-4] and its electrocardiographic correlates are very rapid (>350 beat per minute), irregular in timing, irregular in morphology undulations of the ECG baseline irregularly punctuated by QRS complexes representing ventricular activation after frequency filtration by the AV node. The mechanism of atrial flutter is single-wave macro-reentry [3-5] and its electrocardiographic correlates are rapid (250-350 beat per minute), regular in timing, regular in morphology undulations of the ECG baseline regularly or irregularly punctuated by QRS complexes representing ventricular activation after frequency filtration by the AV node. The mechanism of a true atrial tachycardia is either abnormal automaticity or micro-reentry [6,7] and its electrocardiographic correlates are rapid (100-250 beats per minute), regular or irregular in timing, abnormal p-waves with intervening isoelectric periods regularly or irregularly punctuated by QRS complexes representing ventricular activation after frequency filtration by the AV node. These arrhythmias are facilitated by atrial trauma, stretch, ischemia, epicardial inflammation, hypoxia, acidosis, electrolyte disturbances, and the refractoriness changes that accompany sympathetic nervous system discharge. As all of these factors are frequent immediately after cardiac surgery, it is not surprising that atrial tachyarrhythmias are frequent complications of these procedures. Indeed, atrial tachyarrhythmias are the most common post-operative complication of cardiac surgical procedures that require intervention or prolong hospital stay. The purpose of this review is to take a meta-analytic approach to the wealth of published data regarding the incidence, timing and outcomes of atrial tachyarrhythmias that occur after cardiac surgical procedures.

2. Incidence

Atrial tachyarrhythmias were reported to be a complication of cardiac surgical procedures shortly after their introduction [8]. Of course, the reported incidence of post-operative atrial tachyarrhythmias is very dependent on the characteristics of the patient population studied, the duration of an atrial tachyarrhythmia considered to be important, and the electrocardiographic tools used for screening. As detailed in the following chapter, post-operative atrial tachyarrhythmias are more common in patients with predisposing characteristics or risk factors. These risk factors include older age, a history of atrial tachyarrhythmias, pre-operative atrial dilatation, post-operative elevations in atrial pressures, and withdrawal of pre-operative beta-adrenergic blocking drug therapy. As several of these factors also have multiple etiologies, the list of risk factors for post-operative atrial tachyarrhythmias is long. Patient populations with more of these risk factors will have a higher incidence of post-operative atrial tachyarrhythmias. Published reports of the incidence of post-operative atrial tachyarrhythmias have also used different definitions as to what constitutes an atrial tachyarrhythmia episode that should be considered to be a post-operative complication. At one extreme, a post-operative atrial tachyarrhythmia was considered to have occurred if any electrocardiographic documentation of an atrial tachyarrhythmia was acquired and, at the other extreme, a post-operative atrial tachyarrhythmia was considered to have occurred only if a sustained atrial tachyarrhythmia required treatment or prolonged hospital stay. Finally, the incidence of post-operative atrial tachyarrhythmias also depends on the electrocardiographic tool used to document its occurrence. Clearly, continuous electrocardiographic monitoring with automatic arrhythmia detection algorithms will detect a post-operative atrial tachyarrhythmia more frequently than will ad hoc standard 12-lead electrocardiograms performed when a patient describes symptoms compatible with an atrial tachyarrhythmia. These differences in patient populations studied, definitions of atrial tachyarrhythmias used, and electrocardiographic surveillance methods employed are responsible for the disparate reports of the incidence of post-operative atrial tachyarrhythmias. Nevertheless, by taking a meta-analytic approach to these reports a reasonable estimate of the incidence of post-operative atrial tachyarrhythmias in an average patient population undergoing cardiac surgery should emerge.

2.1. Atrial tachyarrhythmias after coronary bypass surgery

The best studied patient population from the standpoint of the incidence of post-operative atrial tachyarrhythmias is that undergoing isolated coronary artery bypass surgery. Insights into the incidence of post-operative atrial tachyarrhythmias in this patient population are provided by examination of the control groups of the randomized clinical trials that have evaluated prophylactic therapy for post-operative atrial tachyarrhythmias and by examination of large observational reports of patients having coronary artery bypass surgery.

2.1.1. **Lessons from randomized clinical trials.** This analysis considers the control patient populations reported from forty randomized clinical trials [9-48] of prophylactic therapy for post-operative atrial tachyarrhythmias in patients undergoing isolated coronary artery bypass surgery. By definition, these clinical trials collected information relative to the incidence of post-operative atrial tachyarrhythmias in a prospective manner.

Table 1. Incidence of atrial tachyarrhythmias after coronary artery bypass surgery in the control populations of forty randomized clinical trials.

Author	Reference	Year	Active Treatment	Total Control pts (#)	Control pts with AT (#)	Control pts with AT (%)
Davidson	9	1985	verapamil	100	23	23%
Williams	10	1985	verapamil	71	19	27%
Smith	11	1985	verapamil	47	5	11%
Johnson	12	1976	digoxin	66	17	26%
Tyras	13	1979	digoxin	79	9	11%
Weiner	14	1986	digoxin	51	6	12%
Mills	15	1983	dig and prop	90	30	34%
Ormerod	16	1984	dig or prop	33	9	27%
Rubin	17	1987	dig or prop	40	15	38%
Salazar	18	1979	propranolol	22	1	5%
Stephenson	19	1980	propranolol	136	24	18%
Mohr	20	1981	propranolol	48	19	40%
Silverman	21	1982	propranolol	50	14	28%
Williams	22	1982	propranolol	32	6	19%
Abel	23	1983	propranolol	50	19	38%
Ivey	24	1983	propranolol	56	9	16%
Hammon	25	1984	propranolol	26	15	58%
Myhre	26	1984	propranolol	20	9	45%
Matangi	27	1985	propranolol	82	19	23%
Martinussen	28	1988	propranolol	40	5	13%
White	29	1984	timolol	20	19	95%
Vecht	30	1986	timolol	66	13	20%
Materne	31	1985	acebutolol	39	13	33%
Daudon	32	1986	acebutolol	50	20	40%
Khuri	33	1987	nadolol	74	35	42%
Lamb	34	1988	atenolol	30	10	33%
Matangi	35	1989	atenolol	35	26	74%
Janssen	36	1986	sot or meto	50	18	36%
Suttorp	37	1991	sotalol	150	46	31%
Pfisterer	38	1997	sotalol	110	47	43%
Honloser	39	1991	amiodarone	38	8	21%
Butler	40	1993	amiodarone	60	12	20%
Daoud	41	1997	amiodarone	60	25	42%
Redle	42	1997	amiodarone	64	20	31%

Table 1. Continued

Author	Reference	Year	Active Treatment	Total Control pts (#)	Control pts with AT (#)	Control pts with AT (%)
Laub	43	1993	procainamide	24	9	38%
Gold	44	1996	procainamide	50	19	38%
Fanning	45	1991	magnesium	50	14	28%
Parikka	46	1993	magnesium	71	17	24%
Nurozler	47	1996	magnesium	25	5	20%
Klemperer	48	1996	T3	65	21	32%
OVERALL				2270	670	30%

Abbreviations: AT = atrial tachyarrhythmias, dig = digoxin, meto = metoprolol, prop= propranolol, pts = patients, sot = sotalol, T3 = triiodothyronine

The individual estimates of the incidence of atrial tachyarrhythmias after coronary artery bypass surgery reported by these clinical trials ranged range from 5% [18] to 95% (29). Overall, 670 patients (30%) of the 2270 patients in the combined control patient population of these trials experienced this post-operative complication. The 95% confidence interval limits around this point estimate of the incidence of post-operative atrial tachyarrhythmias are 25%-35%.

2.1.2. Lessons from large observational study reports. Reliable estimates of the incidence of atrial tachyarrhythmias after coronary artery bypass surgery may also be found in reports [49-54] of large cohorts of patients observed for this purpose.

Table 2. Incidence of atrial tachyarrhythmias after coronary artery bypass surgery in the populations of six large observational studies.

Author	Reference	Year	Study	Total pts (#)	Pts with AT (#)	Pts with AT (%)
Fuller	49	1989	single-center	1666	473	28%
Leitch	50	1990	single-center	5807	999	17%
Creswell	51	1993	single-center	2833	905	32%
Mathew	52	1996	multi-center	2048	526	26%
Aranki	53	1996	single-center	570	189	33%
Almassi	54	1997	multi-center	3126	863	28%
OVERALL				16,050	3,955	25%

Abbreviations: AT=atrial tachyarrhythmias, pts = patients

The individual estimates of the incidence of atrial tachyarrhythmias after coronary artery bypass surgery reported by these large observational studies ranged from 17% (50) to 33% [53]. Overall, 3,955 patients (25%) of the 16,050 patients in the combined patient populations of these observational reports experienced this post-operative complication. The 95% confidence interval limits around this point estimate of the incidence of post-operative atrial tachyarrhythmias are 20%-30%. This 95% confidence interval overlaps that of the point estimate derived from the control patient populations of the randomized clinical trials.

2.1.3. Combined analysis. The mean incidence of post-operative atrial tachyarrhythmias reported from the control groups of the randomized clinical trials is slightly higher than that from the large observational study reports. This difference likely results from the practice of withdrawing pre-operative beta-blocker drug therapy from patients in the control arms of the randomized clinical trials (contributing to an inflation of the incidence of atrial tachyarrhythmias in this group) [21,23] and the practice of continuing pre-operative beta-blocker drug therapy in patients in the large observational studies (contributing to a deflation of the incidence of atrial tachyarrhythmias in this group) [49,52]. Accordingly, the true incidence of atrial tachyarrhythmias after coronary artery bypass surgery during the period covered by these investigations was likely to be slightly lower than the mean incidence reported from the randomized clinical trials and slightly higher than the mean incidence reported by the large observational studies (in the range of 25%-30%). Nevertheless, the majority of the reports contributing to this analysis are now dated. Over the past two decades, the patient population undergoing coronary artery bypass surgery has changed dramatically. Such patients are now older, have more severe structural heart disease, and have a higher prevalence of comorbid conditions. These population changes have resulted in an increase in the incidence of post-operative atrial arrhythmias [51,53]. Between 1986 and 1991 the incidence of post-operative atrial tachyarrhythmias after coronary artery bypass surgery increased from 26% to 36% at Barnes Hospital in St. Louis [51] and between 1970 and 1992 the incidence of post-operative atrial tachyarrhythmias increased from 5% to 33% at the Brigham and Women's Hospital in Boston [53]. These considerations suggest that the contemporary probability of a post-operative atrial tachyarrhythmia complicating coronary artery bypass surgery is approximately 30%.

2.2. Atrial tachyarrhythmias after valvular heart surgery

The population of patients undergoing valve replacement or valve repair surgery with or without concomitant coronary artery bypass surgery have not been evaluated in randomized clinical trials of prophylactic therapy for atrial tachyarrhythmias in sufficient numbers to properly evaluate the incidence of this post-operative complication. Thus, estimates of the incidence of post-operative atrial tachyarrhythmias in patients undergoing valve replacement or valve repair surgery must be derived from the large observational studies. These studies indicate that patients undergoing valve replacement or valve repair surgery have a higher incidence of post-operative atrial tachyarrhythmias than do patients undergoing isolated coronary artery bypass surgery.

Table 3. Incidence of atrial tachyarrhythmias after valvular heart surgery and after combined coronary artery bypass surgery/valvular heart surgery in the populations of three large observational studies.

Author	Reference	Year	Total valve pts (#)	Pts with AT (%)	Total CABG-valve pts (#)	Pts with AT (%)
Creswell	51	1993	297	48%	273	63%
Mathew	52	1996	--	--	217	42%
Almassi	54	1997	272	35%	263	40%
OVERALL			569	42%	753	49%

Abbreviations: AT=atrial tachyarrhythmias, CABS = coronary artery bypass surgery, CABS-valve = combined CABS and valve surgery procedures, pts = patients, valve = isolated valve surgery

Thus, patients undergoing isolated coronary artery bypass surgery have an average incidence of post-operative atrial tachyarrhythmias of approximately 30%, patients having isolated valvular surgery have an average incidence of post-operative atrial tachyarrhythmias of approximately 40%, and patients having both types of surgical procedures have an average incidence of post-operative atrial tachyarrhythmias of approximately 50%.

3. Timing

3.1. Atrial tachyarrhythmias after coronary bypass surgery

Post-operative atrial fibrillation may occur at any time during the traditional 30-day post-operative period during which new cardiac events are usually ascribed to a complication of the operative procedure. Nevertheless, the vast majority of episodes of atrial fibrillation attributable to cardiac surgery occur within the first week – with a peak incidence between the second and fourth post-operative day. Fifteen of the forty randomized clinical trials that assessed therapy for the prevention of atrial tachyarrhythmias after coronary artery bypass surgery reported the timing of this post-operative complication [10-13,15,19-21,27,32,34,36-38,48]. These fifteen clinical trials presented timing data from 318 patients from their respective control groups who developed post-operative atrial tachyarrhythmias. Two of the large observational studies provided data regarding the timing of the onset of post-operative atrial tachyarrhythmias after coronary artery bypass surgery

[49,53]. These two large observational reports presented data from 662 patients who developed post-operative atrial tachyarrhythmias. Thus, these studies provide data relative to the timing of onset of post-operative atrial tachyarrhythmias from a total of 980 patients.

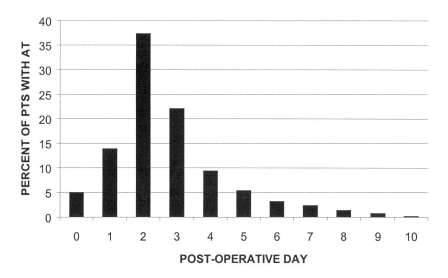

Figure 1. Frequency distribution of day of onset of atrial tachyarrhythmias in 980 patients with post-operative atrial tachyarrhythmias.

The peak incidence of post-operative atrial tachyarrhythmias is on the second post-operative day with over one-third (37%) of such episodes occurring on that day. The days with the next highest incidence of atrial tachyarrhythmias are the contiguous post-operative days one and three. Seventy-three percent of patients who experience a post-operative atrial tachyarrhythmia do so between post-operative days one and three. Of patients destined to experience post-operative atrial tachyarrrhythmias, 87% will do so by the end of the fifth post-operative day.

3.2. Atrial tachyarrhythmias after valvular heart surgery

The data regarding the timing of atrial tachyarrhythmias in patients after valvular heart surgery are much more scant than those in patients after coronary artery bypass surgery. Indeed, they are practically nonexistent. On the other hand, there is no theoretical reason to suspect that the frequency distribution of day of onset of atrial tachyarrhythmias in a valve surgery patient population would be different from that presented above for the coronary artery bypass surgery patient population.

4. Consequences

Post-operative atrial tachyarrhythmias may be of no significance. For example, a transient episode of an atrial tachyarrhythmia with a controlled ventricular response rate in an asymptomatic patient may have no impact on the patient's subsequent post-operative course. Alternatively, a post-operative atrial tachyarrhythmia may express any of the consequences that have been described in other patient settings. In addition to patient discomfort and anxiety, these consequences those related to the effects of a rapid and irregular ventricular response rate, to hemodynamic compromise, to thromboembolic events including stroke, and to the risks of exposure to antiarrhythmia treatments [51-58].

Many, but not all, of the patients who experience post-operative atrial tachyarrhythmias will report associated symptoms. Even in the absence of an evident complication of the atrial arrhythmia these symptoms typically include palpitations, dyspnea, worsening of "post-operative" chest pain, and anxiety. Furthermore, if the atrial tachyarrhythmia produces complications of its own, symptoms related to one or more of the complications may emerge. These complications include precipitation of myocardial ischemia and precipitation of pump failure. Patients convalescing from a cardiac surgical procedure may be more prone to these complications than are patients in the general population because their cardiac status is already compromised and because the post-operative atrial tachyarrhythmia is often associated with a very rapid ventricular response rate secondary to the sympathetic discharge state that occurs after cardiac surgery. Of course, an atrial tachyarrythmia that produces myocardial ischemia or pump failure constitutes a medical emergency. Finally, atrial tachyarrhythmias may be complicated by thromboembolic events. Clot formed within a non-contracting atrium may embolize anywhere with disastrous consequences. Of these, stoke is the most common.

Determination of the frequency of these potential consequences of an atrial tachyarrhythmia is complicated by the need to separate association from causation. Those patients who are the most severely compromised are not only the most likely to develop an atrial tachyarrhythmia but are also the most likely to experience other complications whether or not atrial fibrillation occurs. Therefore, the excess risk of complications that can be attributed to an atrial tachyarrhythmia cannot be confidently defined. Nevertheless, large observational studies have provided data associating post-operative atrial tachyarrhythmias with a wide variety of potential consequences – stroke, congestive heart failure, post-operative myocardial infarction, VT/VF, and permanent pacemaker requirement. Furthermore, patients whose post-operative course is complicated by an atrial tachyarrhythmia require longer hospital stays and generate increased hospital costs.

The magnitude of these associations may be estimated from the combined results of the large observational studies. From a total sample of 10,673 patients undergoing cardiac surgery, significantly more patients with post-operative atrial tachyarrhythmias had a cerebrovascular accident than did patients without post-operative atrial tachyarrhythmias (4.7% versus 1.9%, odds ratio 2.5, 95% CI for odds ratio 2.0-3.2) [51-54]. Similarly, from a total sample of 6,690 patients undergoing cardiac surgery significantly more patients with post-operative atrial tachyarrhythmias had progressive congestive heart failure than did patients without post-operative atrial tachyarrhythmias (6.4% versus 3.4%, odds ratio 1.9, 95% CI for odds ratio 1.5-2.4) [52-54]. From a total sample of 4,425 patients significantly more patients with post-operative atrial tachyarrhythmias had a peri-operative myocardial infarction than did patients without post-operative atrial tachyarrhythmias (5.3% versus 3.0%, odds ratio 1.8, 95% CI for odds ratio 1.3-2.4) [53,54]. A total sample of 4,553 patients indicated that patients with post-operative atrial tachyarrhythmias are also more likely to require a permanent pacemaker implantation (3.6% versus 1.7%, odds ratio 2.2, 95% CI for odds ratio 1.5-3.2) and to experience post-operative ventricular tachycardia or ventricular fibrillation (9.3% versus 4.0%, odds ratio 2.4, 95% CI for odds ration 1.8-3.0) [51,53]. Finally, a total sample of 8,408 patients suggested that patients with post-operative atrial tachyarrhythmias have a higher operative mortality than do those without atrial tachyarrhythmias (5.2% versus 4.1%, odds ratio 1.3, 95% CI for odds ratio 1.0-1.6) [51,53,54].

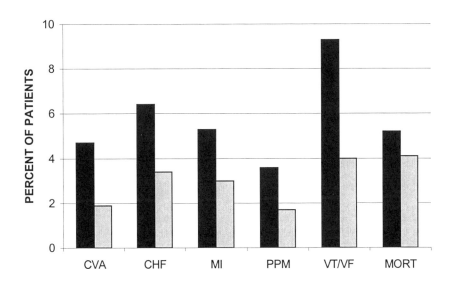

Figure 2. Percentage of patients with post-operative adverse events comparing patients who had post-operative atrial tachyarrhythmias (dark bars) and patients who did not have post-operative atrial tachyarrhythmias (light bars) [references 51-54]. Adverse events: CVA = cerebrovascular accident, CHF = worsening congestive heart failure, MI = myocardial infarction, PPM = permanent pacemaker implantation, VT/VF = ventricular tachycardia/ventricular fibrillation, MORT = operative mortality.

Given the association between post-operative atrial tachyarrhythmias and this wide range of potential adverse consequences, patients with post-operative atrial tachyarrhythmias would also be expected to have longer hospital stays than patients without post-operative atrial tachyarrhythmias. Evidence that this is so is provided by the combined results of three large observational studies [51,52,54] that included a total of 10,673 patients. The lengths of the intensive care unit stay and of the ward stay for patients with post-operative atrial tachyarrhythmias were both significantly longer than those of patients without post-operative atrial tachyarrhythmias (4.4 days versus 2.6 days and 9.0 versus 6.6 days, respectively). These differences translate into a longer total hospital stay for patients with post-operative atrial tachyarrhythmias compared to those without post-operative atrial tachyarrhythmias (13.3 days versus 9.1 days).

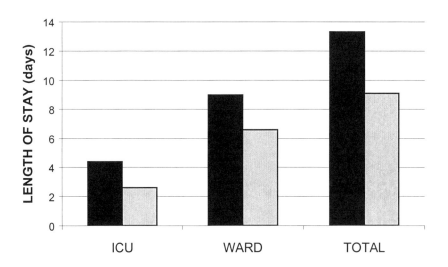

Figure 3. Lengths of hospital stay comparing patients who had post-operative atrial tachyarrhythmias (dark bars) and patients who did not have post-operative atrial tachyarrhythmias (light bars) [references 51,53,54].

Of course, the longer length of stays required to care for patients with post-operative atrial tachyarrhythmias result in an increased cost to provide this care. Estimates of this increased cost have ranged from $1,616 to $10,050 per patient for those undergoing isolated coronary artery bypass surgery [52,54]. If we accept the greater of these estimates and accept that 30% of the 400,000 patients undergoing coronary artery bypass surgery each year in the United States will develop post-operative atrial tachyarrhythmias, the cost of this post-operative complication exceeds 1 billion dollars annually.

5. Conclusions

Post-operative atrial tachyarrhythmias are the most frequent complication of cardiac surgical procedures occurring in approximately 30% of patients having isolated coronary artery bypass surgery, in approximately 40% of patients having isolated valvular heart surgical procedures, and in approximately 50% of patients having both coronary artery bypass and valvular heart surgical procedures. The peak incidence of post-operative atrial tachyarrhythmias is on the third post-operative day with almost 90% of patients destined to experience an atrial tachyarrhythmia doing so by the end of the fifth post-operative day. Post-operative atrial tachyarrhythmias are associated with an increased probability of other post-operative complications including cerebrovascular accidents, worsening congestive heart failure, perioperative myocardial infarction, and operative mortality. Furthermore, post-operative atrial tachyarrhythmias prolong the hospital stay of these patients and increase the cost of provision of revascularization services. The incremental cost of attributable to atrial tachyarrhythmias after cardiac surgery in the United States may be as high as one billion dollars per year.

References

1. Pritchett ELC: Management of atrial fibrillation. N Engl J Med 1992;326:1264-1.
2. Moe GK: On the multiple wavelet hypothesis of atrial fibrillation. Arch Int Pharmacodyn Ther 1982;140:183-8.
3. Allessie M, Lammers W, Smeets J, et al: Total mapping of atrial excitation during acetylcholine-induced atrial flutter and fibrillation in the isolated canine heart. In, Kulbertus HE, Olsson SB, Schlepper M, editors. Atrial Fibrillation. Molndal, Sweden: AB Hasses, 1982;44-59.
4. Cox JL, Canaven TE, Schuessler RB, et al: The surgical treatment of atrial fibrillation. II. Intraoperative electrophysiologic mapping and description of the electrophysiologic basis of atrial flutter and atrial fibrillation. J Thorac Cardiovasc Surg 1991;101:406-426.
5. Olshansky B, Wilber DJ, Hariman RJ: Atrial flutter – update on the mechanism and treatment. PACE 1992;15:2308-35.
6. Haines DE, DiMarco JP. Sustained intraatrial reentrant tachycardia: clinical, electrocardiographic and electrophysiologic characteristics and long-term follow-up. J Am Coll Cardiol 1990;15:1345-54.
7. Chen S-A, Chiang C-E, Yang C-J, et al. Sustained atrial tachycardia in adult patients. Electrophysiological characteristics, pharmacological response, possible mechanisms, and effects of radiofrequency ablation. Circulation 1994;90:1262-78.
8. Favalaro RG, Effler DB, Groves LK, et al. Direct myocardial revascularization with saphenous vein autograft. Dis Chest 1969;56:279-283.
9. Davidson R, Hartz R, Kaplan K, Parker M, Feiereisel P, Michaelis L. Prophylaxis of supraventricular tachyarrhythmia after coronary bypass surgery with oral verapamil: a randomized, double-blind trial. Ann Thorac Surg 1985;39:336-9.
10. WilliamsDB, Misbach GA, Kruse AP, Ivey TD. Oral verapamil for prophylaxis of supraventricular tachycardia after myocardial revascularization. J Thorac Cardiovasc Surg 1985;90:592-6.
11. Smith EEJ, Shore DF, Monro JL, Ross JK. Oral verapamil fails to prevent supraventricular tachycardia following coronary artery surgery. Int J Cardiol 1985;9:37-44.

12. Johnson LW, Dickstein RA, Fruehan T, et al. Prophylactic digitalization for coronary artery bypass surgery. Circulation 1976;53:819-22.

13. Tyras DH, Stothert JC, Kaiser GC, et al. Supraventricular tachyarrhythmias after myocardial revascularization: a randomized trial of prophylactic digitalization. J Thorac Cardiovasc Surg 1979;77:310-4.

14. Weiner B, Rheinlander HF, Decker EL, Cleveland RJ. Digoxin prophylaxis following coronary artery bypass surgery. Clin Pharm 1986;5:55-8.

15. Mills SA, Poole GV Jr, Breyer RH, et al. Digoxin and propranolol in the prophylaxis of dysrhythmias after coronary artery bypass grafting. Circulation 1983;68:II-222 – II-225.

16. Ormerod OJM, McGregor CGA, Stone DL, Wisbey C, Petch MC. Arrhythmias after coronary bypass surgery. Br Heart J 1984;51:618-21.

17. Rubin DA, Nieminski KE, Reed GE, Herman MV. Predictors, prevention, and long-term prognosis of atrial fibrillation after coronary artery bypass graft operations. J Thorac Cardiovasc Surg 1987;94:331-5.

18. Salazar C, Frishman W, Friedman S, et al. β-Blockade therapy for supraventricular tachyarrhythmias after coronary surgery: a propranolol withdrawal syndrome? Angiology 1979;30:816-9.

19. Stephenson LW, LW, MacVaugh H, Tomasello DN, Josephson ME. Propranolol for prevention of postoperative cardiac arrhythmias: a randomized study. Ann Thorac Surg 1980;29:113-6.

20. Mohr R, Smolinsky A, Goor DA. Prevention of supraventricular tachyarrhythmia with low-dose propranolol after coronary bypass. J Thorac Cardiovasc Surg 1981;81:840-5.

21. Silverman NA, Wright R, Levitsky S. Efficacy of low-dose propranolol in preventing postoperative supraventricular tachyarrhythmia. A prospective randomized trial. Ann Surg 1982;196:194-7.

22. Williams JB, Stephanson LW, Holford FD, Langer T, Dunkman B, Josephson ME. Arrhythmia prophylaxis using propranolol after coronary artery surgery. Ann Thorac Surg 1982;34:435-8.

23. Abel RM, van Gelder HM, Liguori J, Gielchinsky I, Parsonnet V. Continued propranolol administration following coronary bypass surgery. Antiarrhythmic effects. Arch Surg 1983;118:727-31.

24. Ivey MF, Ivey TD, Bailey WW, Williams DB, Hessel EA II, Miller DW Jr. Influence of propranolol on supraventricular tachycardia early after coronary artery revascularization. J Thorac Cardiovasc Surg 1983;85:214-8.

25. Hammon JW Jr, Wood AJJ, Prager RL, Wood M, Muirhead J, Bender HW Jr. Perioperative beta blockade with propranolol: reduction in myocardial oxygen demands and incidence of atrial and ventricular arrhythmias. Ann Thorac Surg 1984;38:363-7.

26. Myhre ESP, Sørlie D, Aarbakke J, Hals PA, Straume B. Effects of low dose propranolol after coronary bypass surgery. J Cardiovasc Surg 1984;25:348-52.

27. Matangi MF, Neutze JM, Graham KJ, Hill DG, Kerr AR, Barratt-Boyes BG. Arrhythmia prophylaxis after aorta-coronary bypass. The effect of minidose propranolol. J Thorac Cardiovasc Surg 1985;89:439-43.

28. Martinussen HJ, Lolk A, Szczepanski C, Alstrup P. Supraventricular tachyarrhythmias after coronary bypass surgery: a double blind randomized trial of prophylactic low dose propranolol. Thorac Cardiovasc Surg 1988;36:206-7.

29. White HD, Antman CBE, Glysnn MA, et al. Efficacy and safety of timolol for prevention of supraventricular tachyarrhythmias after coronary artery bypass surgery. Circulation 1984;70:479-84.

30. Vecht RJ, Nicolaides EP, Ikweuke JK, Liassides C, Cleary J, Cooper WB. Incidence and prevention of supraventricular tachyarrhythmias after coronary bypass surgery. Int J Cardiol 1986;13:125-34.

31. Materne P, Larbuisson R, Collignon P, Limet R, Kulbertus H. Preve tion by acebutolol of rhythm disorders following coronary bypass surgery. Int J Cardiol 1985;8:275-83.

32. Daudon P, Corcos T, Gandjbakhch I, Levasseur J-P, Cabrol A, Cabrol C. Prevention of atrial fibrillation by acebutolol after coronary bypass grafting. Am J Cardiol 1987;58:933-6.

33. Khuri SF, Okike N, Josa M, et al. Efficacy of nadolol in preventing supraventricular tachycardia after coronary bypass grafting. Am J Cardiol 1987;60:51D-58D.

34. Lamb RK, Prabhakar G, Thorpe JAC, Smith S, Norton R, Dyde JA. The use of atenolol in the prevention of supraventricular arrhythmias following coronary artery surgery. Eur Heart J 1988;9:32-6.

35. Matangi MF, Strickland J, Garbe GJ, et al. Atenolol for the prevention of arrhythmias following coronary artery bypass grafting. Can J Cardiol 1989;5:229-34.

36. Janssen J, Loomans L, Harink J, Taams M, Brunninkhuis L, van der Starre P, Koostra G. Prevention and treatment of supraventricular tachycardia shortly after coronary artery bypass grafting: a randomized open trial. Angiology 1986;**601-9.**

37. Suttorp MJ, Kingma JH, Peels HOJ, et al. Effectiveness of sotalol in preventing supraventricular tachyarrhythmias shortly after coronary artery bypass grafting. Am J Cardiol 1991;68:1163-9.

38. Pfisterer ME, Klöter-Weber UCD, Huber M, et al. Prevention of supraventricular tachyarrhythmias after open heart operation by low-dose sotalol: a prospective, double-blind, randomized, placebo-controlled study. Ann Thorac Surg 1997;64:1113-9.

39. Honloser SH, Meinertz T, Dammbacher T, et al. Electrocardiographic and antiarrhythmic effects of intravenous amiodarone: results of a prospective, placebo-controlled study. Am Heart J 1991;121:89-95.

40. Butler J, Harriss DR, Sinclair M, Westaby S. Amiodarone prophylaxis for tachycardias after coronary artery surgery: a randomized, double blind, placebo controlled trial. Br Heart J 1993;70:56-60.

41. Daoud EG, Strickberger A, Man KC, et al. Preoperative amiodarone as prophylaxis against atrial fibrillation after heart surgery. N Engl J Med 1997;337:1785-91.

42. Redle JD, Khurana S, Marzan J, Bassett N, et al. Prophylactic low dose amiodarone versus placebo to prevent atrial fibrillation in pateints undergoing coronary artery bypass graft surgery. J Am Coll Cardiol 1997;29:289A

43. Laub GW, Janeira L, Muralidharan S, et al. Prophylactic procainamide for prevention of atrial fibrillation after coronary artery bypass grafting: a prospective, double-blind, randomized, placebo-controlled pilot study. Crit Care Med 1993;21:1471-8.

44. Gold MR, O'Gara PT, Buckley MJ, DeSanctis RW. Efficacy and safety of procainamide in preventing arrhythmias after coronary artery bypass surgery. Am J Cardiol 1996;78:975-9.

45. Fanning WJ, Thomas CS Jr, Roach A, Tomichek R, Alford WC, Stoney WS Jr. Prophylaxis of atrial fibrillation with magnesium sulfate after coronary artery bypass grafting. Ann Thorac Surg 1991;52;529-33.

46. Parikka H, Toivonen L, Pellinen T, Verkkala K, Järvinen A, Nieminen MS. The influence of intravenous magnesium sulphate of the occurrence of atrial fibrillation after coronary artery by-pass operation. Eur Heart J 1993;14:251-8.

47. Nurozler F, Tokgozoglu L, Pasaoglu I, Boke E, Ersoy U, Bozer AY. Atrial fibrillation after coronary artery bypass surgery: predictors and the role of MgSO4 replacement. J Cardiac Surg 1996;11:421-7.

48. Klemperer JD, Klein IL, Ojamaa K, et al. Triiodothyronine therapy lowers the incidence of atrial fibrillation after cardiac operations.

49. Fuller JA, Adams GG, Buxton B. Atrial fibrillation after coronary artery bypass grafting. Is it a disorder of the elderly? J Thorac Cardiovasc Surg 1989;97:821-5.

50. Leitch JW, Thomson D, Baird DK, Harris PJ. The importance of age a a predictor of atrial fibrillation and flutter after coronary artery bypass grafting. J Thorac Cardiovasc Surg 1990;100:338-42.

51. Creswell LL, Schuessler RB, Rosenbloom M, Cox JL. Hazards of postoperative atrial arrhythmias. Ann Thorac Surg 1993;56:539-49.

52. Mathew JP, Parks R, Savino JS, et al. Atrial fibrillation following coronary artery bypass graft surgery. Predictors, outcomes, and resource utilization. JAMA 1996;276:300-6.

53. Aranki SF, Shaw DP, Adams DH, et al. Predictors of atrial fibrillation after coronary artery surgery. Current trends and impact on hospital resources. Circulation 1996;94:390-7.

54. Almassi GH, Schowalter T, Nicolosi AC, et al. Atrial fibrillation after cardiac surgery. A major morbid event? Ann Surg 1997;226:501-13.

55. Taylor GJ, Malik SA, Colliver JA, et al. Usefulness of atrial fibrillation as a predictor of stroke after isolated coronary artery bypass grafting. Am J Cardiol 1987;60:905-7.

56. Reed GL III, Singer DE, Picard EH, DeSanctis RW. Stroke following coronary artery bypass surgery. A case-controlled estimate of the risk from carotid bruits. N Engl J Med 1988;319:1246-50.

57. Coplen SE, Antman EM, Berlin JA. Efficacy and safety of quinidine therapy for maintenance of sinus rhythm after cardioversion. A meta-analysis of randomized control trials. Circulation 1990;82:1106-16.

58. Flaker GC, Blackshear JL, McBride R, Kronmal RA, Halperin JL, Hart RG. Antiarrhythmic drug therapy and cardiac mortality in atrial fibrillation. J AM Coll Cardiol 1992;20:527-32.

4 RISK FACTORS FOR THE DEVELOPMENT OF POSTOPERATIVE ATRIAL FIBRILLATION

Frederick A. Ehlert, MD, Dhiraj D. Narula, MD
and Jonathan S. Steinberg, MD,
St. Luke's-Roosevelt Hospital Center and
Columbia University College of Physicians and
Surgeons, New York, NY

1.   Introduction

Atrial fibrillation (AF) is a frequent event following cardiac surgery, occurring in up to 40% of patients [1-5].   The arrhythmia itself is often benign such that its occurrence is sometimes not labeled as a "complication"; even so, postoperative AF is associated with an increased length of hospital stay following cardiac surgery. In addition, the sequellae of postoperative AF can be severe and even life-threatening including hemodynamic compromise and thromboemboli.   As such, a thorough knowledge of the risk factors associated with the development of the arrhythmia is warranted.   Furthermore, it is essential that this understanding include the underlying mechanisms by which these risk factors predispose, and to seek prevention and early treatment of postoperative AF.

Most clinically encountered AF unrelated to cardiac surgery is thought to result from reentry around fixed and/or functional barriers; the same holds true for postoperative atrial arrhythmias.   Fundamental to the understanding of clinical arrhythmias resulting from a reentrant mechanism are the concepts of substrate, the underlying myocardial condition which makes development of the arrhythmia possible, and trigger, which initiates the arrhythmia in a given situation. As such, "risk factors" for the development of postoperative AF may reflect: 1) underlying abnormalities in the atrial substrate that existed preoperatively, (as would be reflected by a preoperative history of AF or hypertension), 2) abnormalities in the atrial substrate that were created by the surgery itself (such as created by valvular surgery or differences in the technique used for atrial cannulation), or 3) influences which increase the presence of potential triggers for the arrhythmia (such as electrolyte abnormalities, increased sympathetic tone or beta-blocker withdrawal). It is in this context of substrate and trigger that this chapter will discuss risk factors for the development of postoperative AF.

2. Preoperative Clinical Risk Factors

Most preoperative clinical risk factors for the development of postoperative AF indicate (or even create) changes in the electrical substrate of the atrial myocardium. As such, the preoperative clinical risk factors most often evaluated are similar to AF unrelated to cardiac surgery.

2.1. Prior atrial fibrillation and other supraventricular arrhythmias

In a general cardiology population, the presence of prior atrial arrhythmias is strongly associated with the subsequent occurrence of AF; as would be expected, this association persists in patients following cardiac surgery. This association likely results from postoperative persistence of preoperative changes in the atrial structural substrate and of sensitivity to the same triggers which made AF possible previously. Other factors, such as the effect of the so-called "electrical remodeling" must also be considered [6, 7].

While patients with prior, preoperative AF are probably at greatest risk for the development of postoperative AF, supporting literature is less than overwhelming for several reasons. Firstly, a careful and precise definition of the term "prior AF" is absent from the literature. For example, patients with chronic AF prior to cardiac surgery would seem more likely to redevelop AF following that surgery. Some studies evaluating predictors of postoperative AF include these patients [8]; other studies clearly exclude these patients from analysis [9]). Unfortunately, most of the published literature fails to offer any definition of the term "prior AF". Secondly, many large trials evaluating predictors of postoperative AF intentionally exclude patients with preoperative arrhythmias [3,10] complicating analysis of its true role as a risk factor. Along these same lines, several other large trials neither explicitly excluded these patients nor did they include prior AF as a preoperative factor being analyzed [11,2].

Of the studies that do analyze the association of preoperative AF and its postoperative development, the largest study is from the Multicenter Study of Preoperative Ischemia Cardiac Surgery (MCSPI) database [80]. In this study, 2417 patients undergoing CABG with or without concomitant valvular surgery were randomly selected from 24 university-affiliated hospitals around the United States. Clinical variables were evaluated utilizing retrospective chart reviews and physician interviews. Of these patients, 332 had "prior AF" defined as "reported in the medical record or interviews" or present on preoperative ECG. 158/332 (48%) with "prior AF" developed AF during their postoperative hospital stay as compared to 457/1933 (24%) without prior AF (P<0.01).

The nature of "prior AF" is at best incompletely characterized in the MCSPI study. In spite of this limitation, this data demonstrates that AF occurring prior to surgery is clearly associated with an increased occurrence of postoperative AF. This finding can be interpreted as demonstrating the important role of pre-existing substrate in the occurrence of postoperative arrhythmias. However, an additional corollary observation can also be made from the MCSPI data: despite the clearly intentioned inclusion of patients with prior AF, only approximately 50% of those patients actually developed postoperative AF. These findings suggest that appropriate preventative therapy may not be futile and should be considered.

Other published reports clearly support the association of preoperative atrial arrhythmias with the occurrence of postoperative AF. Hashimoto et al [13] in a large, single-center study from the Mayo Clinic, demonstrated remarkably similar findings. In this study of 800 consecutive patients undergoing isolated coronary artery bypass grafting (CABG), postoperative AF occurred in 21/47 (45%) patients with "prior atrial arrhythmias" (a term not clearly defined in the manuscript) as compared to 165/749 (22%) without prior atrial arrhythmias (p<0.001). Interestingly, in this same population, the presence of premature atrial beats on preoperative ECG was also associated with an increased risk of postoperative AF. It is not inconceivable that in the appropriate postoperative setting, these premature beats provide the trigger for AF. Other smaller studies [9,14] have suggested similar findings.

2.2. Age

As with AF unrelated to surgery, increasing age is an independent risk factor predictive of postoperative AF. The largest study from Leitch et al [3] included 5807 consecutive patients from a single institution. In this population, the overall rate of postoperative AF was 17.2%. For those patients under age 40 years the prevalence was 3.7%; for those aged 70 years and older the prevalence of AF was 27.7%. These data produced an odds-ratio per 10-year decile of 1.7; thus, for each 10-year increment in age, the risk of AF increased by 70%. Other large trials have demonstrated similar findings. Almassi et al [10], in a population of 3855 predominantly male patients from Veterans Administration Hospitals across the United States, demonstrated an odds ratio of 1.6 for each additional 10 years of age above 50 years (95% confidence intervals: 1.48-1.75, p<0.0001). Likewise, the MCSPI study cited above [8] demonstrated an odds ratio of 1.24 per 5 year increase in age. Aranki et al [12], in a study of 570 consecutive patients from Brigham and Women's Hospital, demonstrated an odds ratio of 2 for age 70 to 80 years old, 3 for age ≥80 years. Multiple smaller studies have also demonstrated a significant association of increasing age to postoperative AF [9, 15-19].

It has been hypothesized that age related changes in the atrial substrate, such as dilatation, myocardial atrophy and fibrosis, decreased conduction velocity, as well as related co-morbidities may explain the association of age with AF [12].

These changes in substrate exist independently of the event of cardiac surgery; as such, the age-related incidence of postoperative AF could theoretically parallel the age-related incidence of AF in the general population.

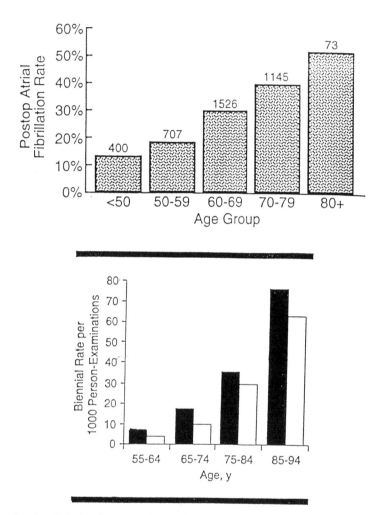

Figure 1. A. Relation between increasing age and postoperative atrial fibrillation as occurring in the PSOCS trial [10], demonstrating the higher rate of postoperative atrial fibrillation in older patients. **B**. Similar age distribution curve for atrial fibrillation occurring in the general population as occurring in the Framingham population [20]. (©American College of Surgery, 1997 and ©1994 American Medical Association. Reproduced with permission).

1 graphically demonstrates this comparison, using the incidence of AF by age in the Framingham population [20] as representative of the general population.   In addition, it is also important to note that direct evidence connecting the above-

described age-related changes in atrial substrate to the age-related increase in ostoperative AF does not exist.

Of note, several small studies have failed to demonstrate an association between age and postoperative AF [14, 21-23]. However, all were studies of 400 or fewer patients and simply compared mean ages of patients with and without postoperative AF.

2.3. Gender

While a strong association between male gender and AF seems well established in the general population, this association remains somewhat more controversial in postoperative AF. For example, large single center trials have reported no association between gender and postoperative AF. Creswell et al [24] evaluated 3983 consecutive patients undergoing cardiac surgery; 1328 (33%) were women. In this study, rates of AF were similar between men and women. In addition, many previously published studies [1,13,19,25-29] have failed to demonstrate an association between gender and postoperative AF when multivariate analysis was performed. However these studies have relatively small numbers of patients and low percentages (10-20%) of women. It is possible that these relatively small samples may be unable to detect differences in rates of AF occurrence relative to gender.

In contrast, two large studies support the association of male gender to postoperative AF. The MCSPI trial [8] included 537 women out of 2417 total patients (24%). In this setting, male gender demonstrated an independent association with AF with an odds ratio of 1.41 (95% confidence intervals: 1.04-1.81). Similarly, Aranki et al [12] with 175 women of 570 total patients (31%) demonstrated a significant association of AF to male gender with an odds ratio of 1.7 (95% confidence intervals: 1.1-2.7). These findings confirm the results of several previously published smaller studies [19, 14, 26]. As a result of these findings, Fuller and co-authors [19] have hypothesized that a hormone-related protective mechanism may account for this gender difference. Others have postulated the existence of hormonal effects on autonomic tone and/or gender differences in 3-dimensional myocardial architecture [8]. These hypotheses remain to be proven.

2.4. Other preoperative medical conditions

Congestive heart failure. The association of a preoperative history of congestive heart failure with the development of postoperative AF is also somewhat controversial. In the MCSPI trial [8], 689 of the 2417 patients (28.5%) had a preoperative history of congestive heart failure defined by ≥NYHA Class II symptoms; of these patients, 238 (35%) developed postoperative AF. In comparison, 24% of patients without prior congestive heart failure symptoms developed postoperative AF. The odds ratio for the association of congestive heart failure with postoperative AF was 1.31 (95% confidence intervals: 1.04-1.64). This association seems plausible given that in the setting of congestive heart failure atrial stretching, thinning, and scarring have been reported; these changes can result in anisotropic conduction, slowing of conduction and dispersion of atrial repolarization. However, in the MCSPI trial, the history of congestive heart failure was determined by a retrospective review of patient records and physician interviews which may in fact have introduced bias. Interestingly, objective measurements associated with congestive heart failure, such as decreased left ventricular ejection fraction and elevated left ventricular end-diastolic pressure, did not predict postoperative AF in this study (see below).

Other large, single center studies have failed to corroborate these findings. Hashimoto et al [13], failed to demonstrate an association between preoperative symptoms of congestive heart failure and postoperative AF; however, in this study elevated left ventricular end-diastolic pressure (>20 mm Hg) was associated with postoperative AF. Likewise, Aranki et al [12] failed to demonstrate an association of previous congestive heart failure to postoperative AF. Several smaller studies have also failed to demonstrate an association [28, 14].

Hypertension. While in the general population the association of systemic hypertension with the development of AF is clearly documented, its association with the development of postoperative AF remains controversial. In data from Leitch et al [3], the largest series to date, postoperative AF developed in 18.2% of patients with a history of hypertension as compared to 16.2% of patients without hypertension (p< 0.05). Almassi et al [10], in a population of 3855 predominantly male veterans, noted a history of hypertension in 702 of the 1143 patients who developed postoperative AF (61.4%); this compared to a history of hypertension in 1571 of the 2711 patients (58%) who did not develop postoperative AF (p=0.046). Resting systolic blood pressure > 120 mm Hg was an independent predictor of postoperative AF in this population. Aranki et al [12], in a single center study, also noted borderline significance to the association of hypertension and postoperative AF: 122/165 (65%) of patients with postoperative AF had previously diagnosed hypertension as compared to 214/381 (56%) of patients without postoperative AF.

Offering conflicting data, the MCSPI trial [8], with 2417 patients from 24 centers, noted a similar incidence of AF in patients with and without a history of hypertension (29% vs. 26%, respectively; p=0.18). Likewise Hashimoto et al [13] demonstrated no association between preoperative hypertension and postoperative AF. Multiple smaller studies have also failed to demonstrate an association [17-19, 22, 26, 28, 30].

Data published from our institution [23] also failed to demonstrate an association between hypertension and postoperative AF; interestingly, however, the presence of left ventricular hypertrophy on the surface ECG was associated with the development of postoperative AF in this same study. Since the ECG changes associated with hypertrophy occur most often in the setting of longstanding hypertension, these findings seem to suggest that changes in the myocardial substrate resulting from hypertension play an important and possibly necessary role in the development of postoperative AF.

Chronic lung disease. The association of preoperative lung disease with the development of postoperative AF is also somewhat controversial with conflicting data present in previously published reports. Almassi et al [10] noted that 219/1141 (19.57%) patients in a Veterans Administration trial who developed postoperative AF had chronic obstructive pulmonary disease (defined as FEV1 <1.5 L); this compared to chronic obstructive pulmonary disease in 367/2714 (13.57%) of patients without postoperative AF. Leitch et al [3], in a series of 5807 consecutive patients, showed a significant association of postoperative AF with "chronic airflow limitation" as defined by "usual clinical criteria". In this series, 25.5% of patients with "chronic airflow limitation" developed postoperative AF as compared to 16.8% without; this difference did not achieve statistical significance. In addition, the MCSPI trial [8] failed to demonstrate and association of with "chronic lung disease" as defined in medical records and physician interviews; further breakdown of the diagnostic category into emphysema, bronchitis or asthma also failed to elucidate an association. Likewise, while Aranki et al [12] demonstrated a trend toward the development of postoperative AF in patients with "chronic lung disease"; this difference failed to reach statistical significance.

Most previously published series have failed to demonstrate a significant association between the development of postoperative AF and the presence of diabetes mellitus [10, 12, 19, 24], history of previous myocardial infarction [3, 8, 10, 19] or prior cardiac surgery [8, 10, 12].

3. Adrenergic Stimulation, Preoperative Beta-Blocker Usage and Beta-Blocker Withdrawal

The sympathetic nervous system has long been hypothesized to play a significant role in the development of AF especially in the postoperative setting [31]. In the experimental and clinical electrophysiology laboratory, adrenergic stimulation has been shown to shorten the refractory period of myocardial tissue [32]. In addition, adrenergic stimulation may increase the frequency of ectopic beats. These changes can have a critical impact on the occurrence of AF [34]. As such, the implication that adrenergic stimulation can provide an adequate trigger for the development of AF has intuitive appeal. It is from this hypothesis that the postoperative use of beta-blocker therapy as a preventative measure for AF had arisen. While this therapy has been extensively studied [1,34-40], the role of adrenergic stimulation, preoperative beta-blocker usage and beta-blocker withdrawal also deserve study. As suggested by Frost et al [35], many postoperative beta-blocker prevention trials fail to account for these effects in control populations.

3.1. Adrenergic stimulation

In the postoperative period, one study has demonstrated an association of increased norepinephrine levels with the occurrence of AF. Kalman et al [18] prospectively studied 131 consecutive patients undergoing coronary bypass surgery of which 65 (50%) developed AF. Serum norepinephrine levels were determined immediately after surgery and every 4 hours for 48 hours following the surgery in sample drawn from the right atrial cavity via a central venous catheter. Patients who developed AF had significantly higher serum norepinephrine levels immediately following surgery (5.78±2.83 nmol/L vs. 3.57±1.31 nmol/L, p<0.0001). In addition, the elevation in norepinephrine levels remained significant for every 4-hour sampling interval in the immediate postoperative period. While this type of sampling represented only generalized sympathetic activity, it clearly documented differences in those patients who developed AF. Not surprisingly, serum norepinephrine levels were significantly higher in those patients on beta-blockers preoperatively. Sun et al [41], studying the effects of hypothermia on the sympathetic response during cardiopulmonary bypass, demonstrated increased norepinephrine, epinephrine and neuropeptide Y levels in patients cooled to 28° C as compared to those cooled to 34° C. Those patients with greater elevations in adrenergic hormones were also more likely to develop postoperative AF.

3.2. Preoperative beta-blocker usage

Several previously published reports have investigated the association of preoperative beta-blocker use with postoperative AF. Leitch et al [3], in the largest study to date, showed that 17.9% of patients on preoperative beta-blockers developed AF as compared to 14.9% not on the medication (p<0.05). In contradistinction, the MCSPI trial [8], in which 42% of the 2417 patients included in the trial were on preoperative beta-blockers, showed no difference in the rates of postoperative AF between the 2 groups. Several smaller studies also demonstrate varying results [14,24]. Important to note, however, is that in none of these studies were the preoperative indications for beta-blocker usage or the postoperative continuation of the drug commented upon. As a result, many of these trials may in fact suggest an association of beta-blocker withdrawal with postoperative AF.

3.3. Postoperative beta-blocker withdrawal

The activation of sympathetic nerves and enhancement of the response to adrenergic stimulation found in the setting of beta-blocker withdrawal can provide the trigger necessary for atrial arrhythmias [18]. In the course of studying the preventative value of postoperative beta-blocker therapy, two studies have specifically investigated the clinical impact of beta-blocker withdrawal in cardiac surgery. Abel et al [37] evaluated 91 patients treated with preoperative propranolol who were randomized to postoperative placebo (withdrawal) or continued propranolol treatment. In the postoperative period with 3 days of continuous telemetry monitoring and symptomatic evaluation thereafter, AF developed in 22/50 (44%) of patients withdrawn from propranolol as compared to 9/41 (22%) of those continued on therapy. In a similarly designed study, Silverman et al [38] demonstrated postoperative AF in 3/50 (6%) of patients (p=0.006) on continued beta-blocker therapy as compared to 14/50 (28%) in the withdrawal group. In addition, White et al [40] and Salazar et al [39] both found two- to five-fold increases in the incidence of postoperative AF when preoperative beta-blocker therapy was discontinued postoperatively. These studies form the basis for the proof of the role of postoperative beta-blocker withdrawal.

4. Preoperative Testing

Diagnostic testing is typically performed for a whole host of reasons prior to cardiac surgery. The diagnostic testing to evaluate the potential for postoperative atrial arrhythmias can: 1) can directly or indirectly evaluate atrial electrical properties by using the surface ECG or signal-averaged P wave, 2) indirectly evaluate and quantitate structural changes in the atrial substrate, such as left atrial size in echocardiography, or 3) indirectly measure extrinsic influences on the atrial substrate, such as heart rate variability measurements for autonomic tone. In general, preoperative diagnostic testing has been disappointing, likely related to the significant impact the actual surgical event must have upon the occurrence of postoperative AF.

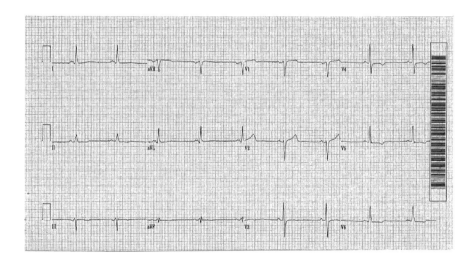

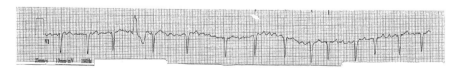

Figure 2A. Preoperative 12-lead electrocardiogram on a 73 year old man undergoing 4 vessel coronary artery bypass surgery. P wave duration is measured at 140 ms. **Figure 2B.** Telemetry monitor strip demonstrating atrial fibrillation on postoperative day 2.

4.1. P wave analysis

The presence of intra-atrial conduction defects on atrial endocardial mapping represents an abnormal electrical substrate. These conduction disturbances have been associated with the occurrence of spontaneous atrial fibrillation [42] and are usually associated with prolongation of the P wave on the surface electrocardiogram [43]. This finding led Buxton and Josephson [44] to first describe the association of preoperative P wave prolongation on the surface ECG and the development of postoperative AF. In their original paper, postoperative AF developed in 24/64 (38%) patients with P wave duration >110 ms as compared to developing in 5/35 (14%) patients with P wave duration ≤110 ms (p<0.05). As such, the technique had a relatively low specificity as a predictive test. In addition, a recent multivariate evaluation (15) has suggested that independent of age and body weight, P wave duration may have little real value. Figure 2 demonstrates a routine preoperative ECG with markedly prolonged P wave duration in a patient who developed AF postoperatively.

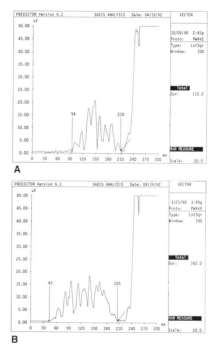

Figure 3. Examples of signal-averaged (SA) P waves. **Top**. SAECG from a patient who did not develop atrial fibrillation (AF) with a measured P-wave duration of 134 milliseconds. **Bottom**. SAECG from patient who had AF on day 3 after coronary bypass graft surgery with a measured P-wave duration of 172 milliseconds. LstSqr indicates least-squares-fit filter; and Proto, protocol. (© American Heart Association, 1993 reproduced with permission).

Signal-averaging applied to the P wave has been used as a more sensitive method for the detection of intra-atrial conduction disturbances [45,46]. Several studies have demonstrated the association of prolonged signal-averaged P wave duration with the development of postoperative AF and the superiority of this technique to P wave duration on the standard surface electrocardiogram [23, 14, 30]. Despite the various signal-averaging methodologies and criteria that have been employed, results have been similarly encouraging. Steinberg et al [23], utilizing a least squares fit filter and a signal-average P wave duration > 140 ms, achieved a sensitivity of 77% and a specificity of 55% for the prediction of postoperative AF. Stafford et al [14], utilizing a spectral analysis filter and signal-averaged P wave duration of >141 ms, achieved similar results in 201 patients. A representative P wave signal-averaged electrocardiogram is presented in Figure 3.

4.2 . Heart rate variability

In an effort to document the association of variations in autonomic tone with postoperative AF, standard assessments of heart rate variability (HRV) have been used. [9,17,47]. All of these studies demonstrated some abnormality in HRV, be it decreased vagal index [9] or "approximate entropy" [47]. However, all studies were performed postoperatively and preoperative data was not available in these patients. Clearly, the intra- and postoperative autonomic state plays an important role in the development of AF (see discussion below). The value of assessing the autonomic state preoperatively remains in question.

4.3. Left atrial size

Relatively few studies [8,13,14] have evaluated the association of increased left atrial size and postoperative AF; none have demonstrated a significant association. The largest numbers are from the MCSPI study [8], which included a subset of 648 patients who underwent preoperative echocardiographic evaluation out of a total 2417 patients in the study. Stafford et al [14] performed preoperative echocardiograms in all 189 patients included in their study. Left atrial diameters were equal (3.6±0.4 cm) in the 51 patients who developed postoperative AF and the 138 who did not.

4.4. Measurements of left ventricular function

While decreased left ventricular function has been associated with the occurrence of AF in the general population, the association following cardiac surgery is less clear. Most problematic in the analysis of this potential association is the variability in assessing left ventricular function and dysfunction. Most studies use left ventricular ejection fraction (LVEF); however, the methodology of determination is often poorly defined if at all. Other studies attempt to use left ventricular end-diastolic pressure determinations, usually those obtained at the time of preoperative angiography. Even these studies fail to account for differences in the time course between data acquisition and surgery.

4.4.1. Cardiomegaly. The simplest and most universally available evaluation of left ventricular dysfunction is the presence of cardiomegaly as evaluated by increased (>0.5) cardiothoracic ratio (CTR) on the standard chest x-ray. Several studies have evaluated the association of this variable with postoperative AF. The largest study, by Leitch et al [3], included 5807 patients from a single center; 20.5% of patients with an increased CTR developed postoperative AF as compared to 16.8% of those without increased CTR (p<0.05). Likewise, the MCSPI database [8], with 2417 patients also showed that an increased CTR was present in 22.7% of patients with AF as compared to 19.8% of those without (p=0.047). However, increased CTR was not an independent predictor of postoperative AF. A smaller study by Stafford et al [14] also failed to demonstrate a significant association of increased CTR with postoperative AF.

4.4.2. Left ventricular ejection fraction. Much of the published data regarding LVEF is at best fragmentary and unavailable for the reader's critical review. In many studies, the method of LVEF determination is poorly defined and not standardized. Analysis often simply divides patients into low and high LVEF groups for simplification of statistical analysis. Finally, many of the published manuscripts fail to present the actual numbers supporting the conclusions.

Nonetheless, most published studies seem to suggest that reduced LVEF is not a preoperative risk factor for postoperative AF. The largest supporting study comes from Fuller et al [2] which included 1666 patients from a single center. In this study LVEF was determined by "single plane ventriculogram"; this variable was reported as not significant in the 473 patients who developed postoperative AF, although no supporting numbers are given. The largest study allowing reader review is from Hashimoto et al [13] in data collected at the Mayo Clinic. Here, LVEF data from cardiac catheterization was obtained in 719 of 800 patients undergoing isolated coronary artery bypass surgery; the LVEF was 57±13% in the 553 patients without postoperative AF as compared to 56±13% in the 166 with postoperative AF. Many smaller studies also support this lack of association between reduced preoperative LVEF and postoperative AF [9,15-18,22,26,30].

However, conflicting data does exist. The largest published series comes from Creswell et al [24] which included 3983 patients from a single center. In this study the LVEF as determined by single plane ventriculogram was 55±17% for the entire cohort of patients. Although LVEF data was available in only "a limited number of patients", the exact number was not specified. "Decreasing [LV]EF" demonstrated a significant association with postoperative AF by univariate analysis; however, multivariate analysis failed to maintain the significance of this association. Likewise, the MCSPI database [8] with 2417 patients also showed that the LVEF was somewhat lower in the patients who developed postoperative AF (52±16% vs. 55±16%, p=0.01); however, LVEF failed as an independent predictor of postoperative AF. Some smaller studies [23,28,48] demonstrate a strong independent association.

4.4.3. Left ventricular end-diastolic pressure. Elevations in left ventricular end-diastolic pressure (LVEDP) are an objective and relatively specific measurement of noncompliant ventricular myocardium; this situation often occurs in the setting of congestive heart failure, ischemia or myocardial hypertrophy. In addition, LVEDP is preoperatively measured in almost all patients at the time of cardiac catheterization and as such, is theoretically useful to predict postoperative AF. Many studies have evaluated LVEDP; most have demonstrated no independent association with postoperative AF. The largest such series, by Leitch et al [3], which defined elevated LVEDP as >15 mmHg, and the MCSPI database [8], which evaluated LVEDP as a continuous variable, demonstrated no association with postoperative AF. Other large series also demonstrated borderline associations of elevations in LVEDP to postoperative AF when analyzed as a continuous variable; however, multivariate analysis failed to maintain the independence of this association [15, 24]. Many smaller series also failed to demonstrate this association [9,18,26].

One large, single-center trial offers an interesting contradiction to these above-noted results. In analysis of 523 patients undergoing isolated coronary artery bypass in whom LVEDP data was available, Hashimoto et al [13] noted no significant difference between the LVEDP of patients who developed postoperative AF and those who did not (19±8 vs. 18±7). However, 80/171 (47%) of patients who developed AF had preoperative LVEDP ≥20 as compared to 216/561 (39%) of patients who did not develop AF. By multivariate analysis, this factor was an independent predictor of postoperative AF.

5. Degree of Preoperative Coronary Artery Disease

The potential association of preoperative coronary artery disease and the development of postoperative AF arose from the hypothetical role of ischemia in the development of AF. This ischemia may be extensive and preoperative, occurring prior to the surgical procedure itself, but creating a damaged atrial myocardial substrate more capable of AF. This ischemia can also be intraoperative, related to the inadequacy of perioperative flow via selective diseased coronary arteries such as the right coronary artery or smaller branch vessels with a more selective distribution of flow to atrial myocardium.

5.1. Extensive coronary artery disease

Relatively few studies have evaluated the association of postoperative atrial fibrillation with the extent of preoperative coronary artery disease. When defined as the >3-vessel and/or left main coronary artery disease, extensive preoperative coronary disease demonstrated some association to postoperative AF in only 2 studies. Leitch et al [3] reported that 18.0% of patients with >3-vessel and/or left main coronary artery disease developed postoperative AF as compared to 15.9% with ≤3-vessel and without left main coronary artery disease (p<0.05); however, multivariate analysis did not support the independence of this association. Frost et al [9] presented similar data in a much smaller population. Several smaller studies with populations ranging from 200 to 800 patients, have also failed to demonstrate any independent association [13, 22, 28].

5.2. Selective coronary artery disease.

Recently, significant interest has arisen regarding the association of significant right coronary artery stenosis with postoperative AF. Studies of patients undergoing non-cardiac surgery have suggested a relationship with myocardial ischemia originating from the right coronary artery [49-51]. Significant right coronary artery stenosis could also limit perfusion of cardioplegia agents into atrial tissue at the time of surgery (see below) suggesting another theoretical etiology for postoperative AF. Based on this reasoning, Mendes et al [26] evaluated right coronary artery stenosis as a predictor of postoperative AF. In a series of 168 consecutive from a single institution, 45/104 patients (43%) with $\geq 70\%$ proximal or mid right coronary stenosis developed postoperative AF. This compared to 12/64 without significant right coronary disease who developed postoperative AF (p=0.001). Multivariate analysis suggested RCA stenosis was an independent predictor of postoperative AF (odds ratio 3.69 [95% CI 1.61-8.48]).

Along these same lines, one small but interesting retrospective study obtained postoperative coronary angiograms comparing patients who developed postoperative AF to those who did not. Interestingly, significant stenosis of the sinoatrial nodal artery was present in 9/25 with postoperative AF as compared to 2/25 without AF (p=0.018); likewise, significant stenosis of the atrioventricular nodal artery was present in 18/25 with postoperative AF as compared to 4/25 without AF (p=0.0001). The presence of disease in these arteries was independently predictive of postoperative AF.

One large, multicenter trial (MCSPI) [8] has subsequently evaluated the association of right coronary artery disease and post operative AF. From this database, 395/1378 (29%) with significant disease developed AF as compared to 222/887 (25%) with our right coronary disease who developed AF (p=0.06). In this trial, multivariate analysis failed to maintain an association. Another smaller study also confirms this lack of association [16].

6. Intraoperative Risk Factors

Keeping with the aforementioned theory of arrhythmia development, technical aspects related to adult cardiac surgery have the potential to create or worsen the atrial myocardial substrate for arrhythmias. For example, the surgical manipulation and exposure required for valvular repair and replacement will affect the atrial arrhythmia substrate to a greater degree than traditional coronary bypass alone. Likewise, other technical factors within the procedure may also affect the substrate as well as create potential triggers for atrial arrhythmias. Since atrial cardioplegia is usually incomplete at best, total procedural time as well as the specifics of cardioplegia techniques can potentially aggravate the risk of AF. In addition, accurate comparisons of these factors are often difficult to make, especially in studies from a single center where single techniques and even a single surgeon may be used in all patients.

6.1. Surgical methodology

Number of coronary artery grafts. The more extensive surgical procedure required to produce multiple coronary artery grafts has been long hypothesized to be a potential factor in the occurrence of postoperative AF. Only one, albeit large, series has supported this belief. Leitch et al [3], in a single-center series including 5807 patients, showed that 18.4% of patients with >3 coronary anastomoses developed postoperative AF; this compared to 16.2% with 3 or fewer coronary anastomoses (p<0.05). In this study, multivariate analysis suggested this surgical factor was an independent predictor for postoperative AF.

No other published series has confirmed this observation, including large, multicenter series. The MCSPI database [8], including 2417 patients from 24 centers, found no difference in the number of grafts between those 617 patients who developed AF and those who did not. Many single-center series including ≥400 patients have also failed to note an association between the number of grafts and postoperative AF: Hashimoto [13], Chew [28], Fuller [19] and Aranki [12] have all shown virtually identical numbers of anastamoses in those patients developed postoperative AF and those who did not. Many smaller single-center series also confirm these findings [16,18,22,26,30]. With the evolution of percutaneous revascularization techniques, most revascularization surgeries now performed include three or more grafts.

Internal mammary artery conduits. A single small study [52] initially suggested that internal mammary artery (IMA) was associated with an increased incidence of postoperative AF. The authors suggested this may be related to pericarditis in the population receiving IMA grafts. Subsequently 2 large multicenter trials have evaluated this association. Aranki et al (AID) in a series of 570 consecutive patients from a single institution found no such association. In this series 155/189 (82%) of patients who developed in hospital AF had internal mammary grafts as compared to IMA grafting in 324/381 (85%) who did not develop AF (p=ns). In contradistinction the MCSPI database, with 2417 patients from 24 institutions, did show some association. Of the 1742 patients with internal mammary grafts 424 (24%) developed AF; this compared to 193/523 (19%) who developed AF in the group with mammary grafts (p<0.01). Multivariate analysis, however, failed to demonstrate an independence to this association.

Minimally invasive direct coronary artery bypass surgery. Significant interest has recently been generated regarding the minimally invasive direct coronary artery bypass (mid-CAB) procedure. Since this procedure is performed without cardiopulmonary bypass and cardioplegia, atrial damage is theoretically less likely to occur. In an extensive review of the mid-CAB literature, only 2 series mention the occurrence of postoperative AF. Subramanian et al [53] notes "clinically significant AF", that is requiring treatment with intravenous medication for ≥24 hours, in 14 of 185 patients undergoing mid-CAB at a single institution. Arom et al [54] reported "new AF" in 13/55 "low-risk" operative patients undergoing mid-CAB; this series also reported postoperative AF in 12/17 patients undergoing mid-CAB who were considered too "high-risk" for conventional CABG procedures. Recently published data from our institution suggests similar rates of postoperative AF when comparing patients undergoing mid-CAB to those undergoing conventional coronary artery bypass procedures [55].

Valvular surgery. The importance of extensive myocardial surgery such as valvular repair or replacement has been extensively investigated as a significant risk factor for the development of postoperative AF in two large studies. The MCSPI database [8] included 217 patients undergoing combined CABG and valvular surgery (or 10% of the total study population); 91 (42%) developed AF during in-hospital follow-up. In comparison, 526/2046 (26%) undergoing CABG alone developed AF (p<0.01). Specifically, 31 of 64 patients (48%) undergoing mitral valve surgery developed AF. However, when multivariate analysis was applied, mitral valve surgery was not an independent predictor for the development of postoperative AF. Several smaller studies report similar findings [23,56].

In contrast, the PSCOS trial [10], including 3855 patients from VA Medical Centers around the US, suggested mitral valve surgery may be an independent risk factor. Postoperative AF developed in 53 of 105 patients (49%) undergoing mitral valve replacement alone or in combination with other cardiac surgery. Postoperative AF also developed in 38 of 72 patients (53%) undergoing mitral valve repair alone or in combination with CABG. Both factors were independent predictors of postoperative AF by multivariate analysis. Of note, and in contradistinction to the MCSPI trial, this VA trial deliberately excluded patients with preoperative AF; this may have resulted in the exclusion of many if not most patients requiring mitral valvular surgery. Most large studies evaluating postoperative AF deliberately exclude patients undergoing valvular surgery from analysis, allowing evaluation of predictive factors only in CABG surgery patients [12,13,19].

6.2. Techniques utilized in cardiopulmonary bypass

Coinciding with the development of cardiac surgery has been the development of techniques for maintaining viability of vital organs and peripheral tissues as well as techniques for minimizing myocardial ischemia during the surgery. Because of these advances, most cardiac surgery today is performed utilizing cardiopulmonary bypass and cardioplegia. Different timing, duration and technique can be used in vascular cannulation and aortic cross-clamping as part of cardiopulmonary bypass. All have the potential to affect the atrial myocardial substrate and to provide triggers for the occurrence of postoperative AF. Again, analysis of these types of variables can prove to be difficult because single surgeons and even single surgical centers tend to consistently use a single technique.

Venous Cannulation Techniques for Establishing Cardiopulmonary Bypass. Significant variability exists in the technique utilized to establish venous access for cardiopulmonary bypass. The most commonly used technique involves cannulation of the inferior vena cava through the right atrial appendage; the catheter utilized for this technique has a basket lying in the right atrium to collect additional right atrial blood returning from the superior vena cava and the Thebesian system. A second approach, called bicaval cannulation, is often used for the more extensive surgeries like valvular repair or replacement, and involves separate catheters cannulating the inferior vena cava via a low right atrial entry and a superior vena cava catheter with traditional entry via the right atrial appendage. These techniques have the potential to create conduction barriers which serve as a substrate for postoperative arrhythmias within the right atrium; as such their role in postoperative AF is intuitively appealing. However few studies have evaluated the clinical impact of various methods of venous drainage. One study [57], a consecutive series at a single center, compared 156 patients with bicaval to 56 with single catheter cannulation and found no significant difference in the occurrence of all types of postoperative atrial arrhythmias. A more recent multicenter study, the MCSPI trial [8], reported AF developing in 112 of 294 patients (38%) with bicaval cannulation as compared to postoperative AF in 489 of 1899 (25%) without ($p<0.01$); this factor remained an independent predictor of postoperative AF on multivariate analysis.

Time on Cardiopulmonary Bypass. Cardiopulmonary bypass is typically established prior to the initiation of cardioplegia and also represents a period of time when the myocardium is faced with potential ischemic compromise. The vast majority of reports in the literature suggest no association between "pump time" and the development of postoperative AF [9,12,13,15-18,23,26,28,30]. Most of these reports are also series of 100+ patients from single surgical centers; these studies present their data as a comparison of mean time on cardiopulmonary bypass pump between patients developing and those not developing postoperative AF. Two large multicenter trials appear to confirm these findings. The PSOCS trial [10], with 3855 patients from 14 VA hospitals around the US, demonstrated no difference in duration of cardiopulmonary bypass undergoing all types of cardiac surgery. A second study, the MCSPI trial, evaluated 2417 patients undergoing cardiac surgery at 24 centers around the US. This study noted a small but significant difference between patients who developed AF and those who did not (median time: 108 vs 99 minutes, $p<0.01$); however, multivariate analysis demonstrated this was not an independent predictor of AF.

Independent of "pump time" and the inherent potential for myocardial ischemia associated with cardiopulmonary bypass, many other physiologic effects may be present and potentially influence the substrate and triggers for atrial arrhythmias. For example, Sun et al [41], studying the effects of hypothermia on the sympathetic response during cardiopulmonary bypass, reported that postoperative AF developed in 8 of 12 patients cooled to 28° C as compared to 2 of 12 patients cooled to only 34° C. Their findings suggested this increased incidence was associated with increased neurohormonal levels in the more hypothermic group.

Aortic Cross-Clamp Time. Most studies of the effect of intraoperative factors on the development of postoperative AF evaluate the aortic cross-clamp time. In most centers, this measurement reflects the period of time of the actual cardiac surgery; that is, after cardiopulmonary bypass and cardioplegia have been established, the period of time when physiologic antegrade blood flow through the coronary arteries has ceased and during which the proximal and distal graft anastomoses are performed. As such, it most precisely reflects the time of greatest ischemic potential for the myocardium.

As with "pump time", the majority of reports in the literature suggest there is no association of aortic cross-clamp time to the development of postoperative AF [9,13-18,23,26,30]. Again, most of these reports are series of 100+ patients from a single surgical center and report mean cross-clamp times ranging from 30 to 60 minutes. The largest of these are reports, studies by Creswell and colleagues [24] from the US and by Fuller et al [58] from Australia, included 2388 and 1666 patients, respectively.

Three additional studies provide conflicting data that warrants further discussion [8,22,28]. The MCSPI database [8], including 2417 patients from 24 centers around the US, demonstrated a 6% increase in the incidence of postoperative AF for each additional 15 minutes of aortic cross clamp time. The overall mean cross-clamp time in this study was not reported. While the actual magnitude of the increase in AF was small, aortic cross-clamp time remained an independent risk factor for postoperative AF when evaluated by multivariate analysis. The two other series, with 400 patients [28] and 200 patients [22], reported considerably longer cross-clamp times for their entire study population (58±11 and 94±41 minutes, respectively), and significantly longer cross-clamp times in those patients who developed AF.

Techniques for Left Ventricular Venting. A variety of venting techniques have been employed during the surgical procedure to reduce the volume of left ventricular blood which can well up and obscure the surgical field following aortic cross-clamp. Vents can be placed in the pulmonary artery to reduce left ventricular filling, via the pulmonary vein, into the left atrium and left ventricle (most commonly via the right superior pulmonary vein), via the aortic root or through the left ventricular apex. The surgical incisions made for placement of these catheters and the sutures necessary for fixation and closure following their removal obviously create potential substrate for postoperative atrial arrhythmias.

The most extensive review of venting techniques comes from the multicenter MCSPI database [8]. In this study, 177 of 525 (34%) patients with pulmonary vein venting developed postoperative AF as compared to 433 of 1710 without this type of venting (p= < 0.01 odds ratio = 1.33[1.15-1.54]). Likewise, 35 of the 92 patients (38%) with left ventricular apex venting developed AF as compared to 575 of 2143 (27%) who did not (p=0.03, odds ratio = 1.42 [1.08-1.86]). Finally, 233 of the 967 (24%) patients with aortic root venting developed AF as compared to 377 of 1268 (30%) without (p<0.01, odds ratio=0.81 [0.70-0.93]). By multivariate analysis, only pulmonary vein venting remained a significant predictor of postoperative AF.

The PSOCS study [10] from Veterans Hospitals across the US reported similar findings. This study evaluated various venting techniques (aorta, right superior pulmonary vein, left ventricular apex and pulmonary artery) for their association with post operative AF. In this study, 35.03% of those patients who developed AF had right superior pulmonary vein venting as compare 25.05% who did not developed AF (p=0.001). Interestingly, 56.54% of patients who developed AF had received aortic venting, while 65.68% who did not develop AF had received it (p=0.001). Also this study noted that this venting technique was used in 5.44% of patients who developed AF and 4.30% of those who did not (p=ns). By multivariate analysis venting via the right superior pulmonary vein remained an independent risk for the development of post-operative AF (p=0.0001, odds ratio = 1.42 [1.21-1.67]).

Mathew and coworkers [8] hypothesize that sudden changes in fiber orientation in combination with surgical scarring from the substrate for arrhythmia in pulmonary vein venting. They point out that in the left atrium little trabeculation exists; however, thicker bundles of atrial muscle exist between and around the orifices of pulmonary veins and venting techniques may selectively injure and disrupt these regions.

6.3. Techniques utilized in cardioplegia

Cardioplegia (literally, paralysis of the myocardium) allows more complete and extensive cardiac surgery and may be helpful in minimizing the potential for ischemic injury. Various methods of establishing and maintaining cardioplegia have been utilized, but for obvious reasons the majority of published work have evaluated the effects of these methods on the ventricular myocardium. On a tissue level, the effectiveness and consequence of cardioplegia in the atria has been investigated. Based on this work, the inadequacy of atrial cardioplegia has been hypothesized to be an important factor in the occurrence of postoperative AF [47]. Nonetheless, direct clinical evidence supporting this hypothesis is far from overwhelming.

While cardiac surgery can be performed without cardioplegia, most centers utilize the technique in some form. As such, a direct comparison of postoperative AF in patients receiving cardioplegia (in any form) versus those receiving none can be difficult. At least one study suggests that cardioplegia may decrease the incidence of postoperative AF. Leitch et al [3], in a series of 4807 patients, showed the rate of AF occurrence was 16.4% in patients receiving cardioplegia versus 17.3% in those not receiving cardioplegia. However, this difference failed to reach statistical significance on multivariate analysis. In this single-center series, only crystalloid cardioplegia was utilized (see below).

Route of cardioplegia administration. The solution establishing cardioplegia can be delivered to the heart by antegrade infusion through the coronary arterial system, by retrograde infusion through the coronary sinus or by a combination of the two. Theoretically, retrograde perfusion of atrial myocardium would be less complete due to the significant role of Thebesian veins in atrial venous return. Likewise, antegrade perfusion of atrial myocardium is theoretically highly dependent on right coronary blood flow (see above).

Several large clinical studies have evaluated the route of cardioplegia administration and its potential role in postoperative AF. The largest study [59], a series of >7000 patients, compared retrograde administration to a combined antegrade/retrograde route. Of the 4224 patients receiving retrograde cardioplegia, 1438 (34%) developed postoperative AF as compared to 880/2808 patients (31%) who received combined antegrade/retrograde cardioplegia (p=0.006). While this study provides strong statistical evidence that retrograde cardioplegia is an independent predictor of postoperative AF, the actual difference demonstrated between the two groups is relatively small.

Other large, multicenter studies evaluating this issue have not demonstrated the same results. The MCSPI database [8] found postoperative AF in 219/735 (30%) patients receiving retrograde cardioplegia as compared to 398/1530 (26%) in those who did not; this difference did not achieve statistical significance (p=0.07).

Cold versus warm cardioplegia. Cardioplegia can be established by chemical means, typically utilizing a solution of low Na^+ and/or high K^+ concentrations. These agents significantly alter the transmembrane potential, resulting in the elimination of mechanical and electrical activity in the myocardium. Cardioplegia can also be established by thermal means, utilizing an infusion of cold solution which significantly lowers myocardial temperatures thereby eliminating mechanical and electrical activity and reducing metabolic needs. Few studies have directly compared the association of these differing methods with postoperative AF.

The PSOCS database [10] seems to suggest that the "method of cardioplegia" is not significant predictor of postoperative AF. In this study, which included 3855 patients, cold antegrade cardioplegia had no effect on the incidence of postoperative AF: 88.3% of patients who developed AF had received cold antegrade cardioplegia as compared to 89.8% who did not develop AF (p=ns). In this study, the use of warm antegrade cardioplegia did show a stronger association: 32.1% of patients developing AF had received it as compared to 28.0% who did not develop AF (p=0.012). However, multivariate analysis failed to establish the independence of this association. No other multicenter trial evaluates these methods directly.

In laboratory studies, Smith et al [60] demonstrated that rapid cooling (to 8°C) of the ventricular septum occurred after initial infusion of cardioplegia solution. However, the atrial septum cooled to only 22° C with the same infusion and rewarmed within 3 - 5 minutes. The comparison of these temperatures over a time course of 10 minutes is demonstrated in Figure 4.

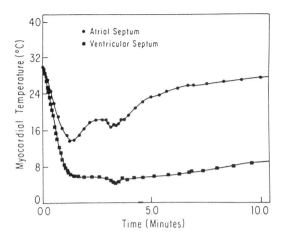

Figure 4. Differences in temperature of the atrial septum and ventricular septum when measured simultaneously and continuously in a patient undergoing routine coronary artery bypass grafting using antegrade cold crystalloid cardioplegia for myocardial preservation. (© Society of Thoracic Surgeons, 1993; reproduced with permission.)

Thus, it is clear that the adequacy of cardioplegia of atrial tissue may at best be variable and atrial ischemic injury resulting from this inadequacy during cardiac surgery may be common. The impact of inadequate atrial cardioplegia on the development of postoperative atrial arrhythmias has not been directly measured.

As a correlate, continued electrical activity has been documented in atrial myocardium following what was thought to be adequate cardioplegia [61]. Tchervenko [62] has shown this activity to correlate with atrial arrhythmias, where as Dewar [63] and Mullen [64] have not. As such, the concept of cardioplegia standstill may not hold for the atria.

The inadequacy of atrial cooling is likely related to more complicated factors than issues of atrial perfusion. During adult cardiac surgery, the right atrium is the most exposed part of the heart. As such, warming from ambient air and operative lighting can be significant. The additional application of topical ice slush may help to maintain atrial cooling and therefore decrease the potential for atrial ischemia. The PSOCS trial [10] also analyzed the addition of topical ice slush to the cardioplegia routine and its association with the development of postoperative AF. Of the patients not receiving topical ice slush, 47.7% developed postoperative AF; this compared to 41.8% receiving topical ice. The absence of ice was found to be an independent predictor of AF (odds ration 1.24, confidence intervals 1.11-1.50, p < 0.001). The same study, however, suggested that topical cold saline had no effect on preventing postoperative AF. Another smaller study [63] also showed 7/12 (58%) patients without topical cooling developed AF as compared to 18/88 (20%) patients with topical cooling (p< 0.02). These series seem to imply that the additional cooling provided by ice slush in fact does prevent postoperative AF.

Blood versus crystalloid cardioplegia. In the cardiothoracic surgical literature, much has been published in an effort to establish the optimal composition of cardioplegia solutions. This discussion includes the relative efficacy of oxygenated blood and unoxygenated (crystalloid) solutions.

Focusing the discussion on the association of cardioplegia solution with postoperative AF does not lessen the controversy. Two published series have specifically examined this issue; both give conflicting results. Rouson et al [57] evaluated consecutive patient groups comparing cold blood to cold crystalloid solution as well as venous drainage techniques. Of the 50 patients receiving cold blood cardioplegia only 2 developed atrial arrhythmias. This compared to rates of atrial arrhythmias varying from 19 to 33% among patients receiving cold crystalloid cardioplegia. This difference was reported as significant p<0.05) and independent of high- or low- volume infusion, high or low K+ concentration and single or double venous catheters. However, multivariate analysis was not performed. The authors suggested that the oxygen provided by blood may be protective but offered no data in support of this hypothesis.

More recently, Pehkonen [27] reexamined this issue in a direct manner controlling for other surgical factors. Postoperative AF developed in 21/49 (43%) patients receiving cold blood cardioplegia as compared to 9/49 (18%) receiving cold crystalloid (p<0.01). Preoperative characteristics were similar between the two groups. Of note, the time to AF onset, number and duration of AF episodes and average heart rate in AF did not differ between the groups. Based on these findings and its contradiction with previously published reports, the authors concluded the vehicle of cardioplegia has less of an effect than does the adequacy of true atrial cardioplegia.

7. Postoperative Factors

Since the development of arrhythmias depends on substrate and trigger, it stands to reason that postoperative atrial arrhythmias are highly influenced by the status of the patient after cardiac surgery. Likely associations exist between postoperative atrial arrhythmias and postoperative complications such as myocardial infarction, heart failure and respiratory difficulties. The mechanisms underlying these associations are multiple; however, the heightened adrenergic stage produced by many complications would seem to play a significant role.

7.1. Serum electrolyte abnormalitie
.

Serum electrolyte levels can over a short period of time vary widely in response to a host of hormonal, pharmacological and membrane factors. For example, following cardiopulmonary by pass and cardioplegia significant changes in serum electrolyte levels, especially potassium, can occur. Upon removal from cardiopulmonary bypass, K^+ levels are typically normalized immediately to between 4.0 and 5.0 mEq/L. Thereafter, treatment with various medications such as pressor agents and diuretics create additional change. As such, significant temporal variation of these measurements exists and resultant attempts to categorize electrolyte abnormalities predictive of postoperative AF may be confusing or even misrepresentative. Relatively few published reports have presented such data.

Potassium. Given its role in cellular depolarization and repolarization, potassium clearly plays a critical role in the development of arrhythmias. The ability of the serum potassium level to reflect or predict the development of cardiac arrhythmias has been discussed for many years [64]. Early reports by Ellis [65] suggested that hyperkalemic cardioplegia solutions played a role in the development of postoperative AF. However subsequent work has failed to substantiate this finding [66].

One paper suggests the association of hypokalemia and postoperative AF. Chew and Ong [28] reported hypokalemia in association with postoperative AF. In their single center series of 400 patients, serum K^+ levels were normalized (4.0-5.0 mEq/L) post-bypass and tested every 4 hours as well as for the occurrence of AF. The authors reported a mean K^+ of 3.6±0.2 mEq/L in the 57 patients with atrial arrhythmias as compared to 4.2±0.3 mEq/L in the 343 with sinus rhythm (p<0.001). However, methodology including timing of K^+ levels used for comparison and calculation of "mean" levels are poorly defined in the text. Kalman [18] reported no difference in serum potassium levels immediately post bypass between patients who developed AF and those who did not.

Magnesium. Magnesium is the second most abundant intracellular cation. Its deficiency has been documented following cardiopulmonary bypass, the result of hemodilution, diuretic use, secondary hypoaldosteronism and the increased anabolic state [16,66,67]. However, relatively few reports have directly investigated the relationship of the serum magnesium level to the development of postoperative AF. Zaman et al [16] evaluated serum Mg^{++} levels preoperatively and on postoperative days 1,2 and 4 in 105 consecutive patients undergoing bypass surgery. While preoperative levels were identical, on postoperative day 1 the 27 patients who developed AF had a serum level of 0.62±0.1 mmol/L as compared to 0.72±0.1 mmol/L in the 74 patients without AF (p<0.001); this difference was an independent predictor of AF. Significant differences were not present in subsequent measurements on days 2 and 4. Kalman et al [18] noted similar but clinically less striking findings in serum Mg^{++} levels measured 24 hours postoperatively (0.79±0.09 mmol/L in patients with AF as compared to 0.83±0.10 mmol/L in patients without AF [p=0.02]). Several studies have been unsuccessful in attempting to prevent postoperative AF using magnesium infusion [68,69,70].

7.2. Postoperative use of pressor and inotropic agents

Two large, multicenter studies suggest the association of the postoperative use of pressor and inotropic agents and the development of AF. In the PSOCS trial including 2417 patients from Veterans Hospitals around the US [10], 66.17% of patients who developed postoperative AF received pressors for >30 minutes following the operation as compared to only 56.00% in the patients without AF (p<0.001). On multivariate analysis, pressor use >30 minutes was an independent predictor of AF with an odds ratio of 1.36 (1.16-1.59). Similar findings were also noted in patients in whom inotrope use persisted for >60 minutes. A few smaller single center studies [23,30] fail to confirm this association.

Mathew et al noted similar results for the use of inotropic agents in the MCSPI database [8]. In this study, 424 of 1454 patients (29%) who received pressor agents postoperatively developed AF as compared to 193 of 803 (24%) who did not develop AF (p=0.01). This difference persisted when patients receiving pressor agents only in the operating room were also included. However, in this study, multivariate analysis failed to demonstrate the independence of the use of inotropic agents as a predictor of postoperative AF.

The use of inotropic agents in the postoperative period is frequently related to the degree of preoperative myocardial dysfunction and to intraoperative events that might result in inadequate myocardial protection. These factors clearly represent a substrate with an increased propensity for postoperative arrhythmias. In addition, the direct and indirect stimulation of myocardial tissue by these agents also provides a potent trigger for these arrhythmias. However, in evaluating this data, one must note that some surgeons routinely use inotropic agents when weaning patients from cardiopulmonary bypass. While both these studies attempt to eliminate such "weaned-only" patients by instituting arbitrary cutoffs of 30 minutes or operating room only, it cannot be known how many such patients were actually included. While little clear-cut data is available, the use of these agents does seem to be associated with the development of postoperative AF.

7.3. Peri- and postoperative myocardial infarction

In a general cardiology population, AF occurs in 10-15% of patients with acute myocardial infarction [67]. As such, it would seem reasonable to expect that perioperative myocardial infarction would be associated with an increased incidence of AF. However, many studies with various sized populations have failed to demonstrate such an association [12,14,15,18,19,22,70]. The largest of these from Fuller et al [19] and Aranki [14] were single institution studies including 1666 and 800 consecutive patients, respectively. The incidence of postoperative myocardial infarction in these series varied between 0 and 10%.

One multicenter trial offered slightly different results. Almassi et al in the PSOCS trial [10] noted perioperative myocardial infarction in 84 of 1133 (7.4%) of patients with postoperative AF as compared to infarction in 91 of 2709 (3.4%) patients without AF (p<0.001). However, the independence of this association was not evaluated along with other potential risk factors, as the authors suggest that infarction may result from the AF rather than the reverse. The authors also correctly caution that interpretation of this information must be tempered. ECG and cardiac enzymes are obtained in almost all patients in whom AF develops, increasing the biased likelihood of diagnosing myocardial infarction.

7.4. Postoperative pericarditis

Pericarditis developing following surgery is frequently discussed as a potential risk factor for the development of postoperative AF. This potential association is intuitively appealing given that sterile pericarditis is used in the animal laboratory to provide a model for mapping studies of AF [71,72]. It also would seem to be supported by the strong association of pericardial irritation and AF in the setting of other thoracic events and surgeries [73,74].

Surprisingly, pericarditis is rarely mentioned in the postoperative AF literature, an absence which may arise from the ubiquitous nature of postoperative pericardial irritation. By definition, all patients undergoing cardiac surgery require pericardial interruption and many patients demonstrate some degree of pericarditis postoperatively. Even more surprisingly, the few studies that exist have failed to support this potential association. Crosby et al [70], in a single center study, noted pericarditis in only 8 of 122 (6.6%) patients who developed postoperative AF as compared to its occurrence in 23 of the 296 (7.8%) who did not (p=ns). In this study, the strict definition of pericarditis ("an audible pericardial friction rub after the removal of all chest tubes" occurring with "associated symptomatology" and requiring treatment with anti-inflammatory agents) limited the number of patients so diagnosed. Using a less strict definition, Rubin and colleagues [1] noted pericarditis in 61 of 123 (50%) total patients in their study of potential risk factors for the development of postoperative AF. Twelve of 36 (33%) patients who developed AF had pericarditis as compared to 49 of 87 (56%) without AF; this difference as not statistically significant.

7.5. Other non-cardiac complications

A postoperative course complicated by respiratory difficulties would also seem likely to be associated with the development of AF. Several large studies have confirmed these suspicions strong associations of postoperative AF with respiratory failure and the need for prolonged ventilator support [12,13,15], the need for reintubation [10,12], and development of pulmonary infiltrates and pneumonia [10,12].

The development of renal failure requiring hemofiltration or dialysis [12, 13] and the development of non-pulmonary nosocomial infections [12,13] have also been associated with higher incidence of postoperative AF. As with evaluation of all postoperative variables and the association with postoperative AF, interpretation must be careful to avoid a "cause-and-effect" mindset. Because the temporal sequence of events is not clear; it is just as possible that AF precipitated the development of further medical complications as is the reverse.

8. Conclusion

The common complication of postoperative AF is, like all arrhythmias, related to the underlying atrial myocardial substrate and conditions which can trigger the arrhythmia. Not surprisingly, many of the same risk factors associated with the development of AF unrelated to the surgical state are associated with its postoperative development. These conditions have preoperatively created an atrial myocardium capable of AF; this substrate is maintained postoperatively. Likewise, the triggers for the arrhythmia often persist into the postoperative state. However, the additional structural and physiological stresses created by cardiac surgery add significantly to the already complicated milieu.

Many potential risk factors for the development of AF following cardiac surgery have been analyzed. Although most make intuitive sense in the context of substrate and trigger, the association of these potential risk factors to AF have varying degrees of support in the published literature. Along this line, Table 1 is included both to summarize the discussions contained in this chapter and to categorize potential risk factors as probable, possible and unlikely based on a review of the literature. The goal of any careful analysis of risk factors for a disease is prospective awareness of potential problems, prevention and the elimination of avoidable risks, and early and aggressive therapy. The same holds true for this analysis of the risk factors for the development of postoperative atrial fibrillation.

Table 1.

Risk Factors Associated With The Development Of Atrial Fibrillation Following Cardiac Surgery.

A. Probable Association
  Preoperative / Clinical Risk Factors
    Prior Atrial Fibrillation
    Advanced Age
    Male Gender
    Prolonged P wave on Signal-Averaged ECG
  Intraoperative / Postoperative Risk Factors
    Postoperative Beta-Blocker Withdrawal
    Bicaval Venous Cannulation for Cardiopulmonary Bypass
    Pulmonary Venous Venting
    Absence of Aortic Root Venting
    Postoperative Use of Pressor Agents

B. Possible Association
  Preoperative / Clinical Risk Factors
    Congestive Heart Failure
    Hypertension
    Chronic Lung Disease
    Prolonged P wave on Surface ECG
    Cardiomegaly on Chest X-ray
    Decreased Left Ventricular Ejection Fraction

Elevated Left Ventricular End Diastolic Pressure
Preoperative Beta-Blocker Use
Intraoperative / Postoperative Risk Factors
Retrograde Cardioplegia
Warm Antegrade Cardioplegia
Serum Hypomagnesemia
Valvular Surgery
Aortic Cross-Clamp Time
Time on Cardiopulmonary Bypass
Cold Crystalloid Cardioplegia
Hyperkalemic Cardioplegia
Postoperative Use of Inotropic Agents
Peri- or Postoperative Myocardial Infarction

C. Unlikely Association

Preoperative / Clinical Risk Factors
Extensive Coronary Artery Stenosis
Right Coronary Artery Stenosis
Intraoperative / Postoperative Risk Factors
Number of Coronary Artery Grafts
Internal Artery Grafts
Minimally Invasive Coronary Artery Bypass
Postoperative Pericarditis

References

1. Rubin DA, Neiminski KE, Reed GE, Herman MV. Predictors, prevention, and long-term prognosis of atrial fibrillation after coronary bypass graft operations. J Thorac Cardiovasc Surg 1987; 94:331-5.2.
2. .Lauer MS, Eagle KA, Buckley MJ, DeSanctis RW. Atrial fibrillation following coronary artery bypass surgery. Prog in Cardiovasc Diseases 1989;31(5):367-378.
3. Leitch JW, Thomson D, Baird DK, Harris PJ. The importance of age as a predictor of atrial fibrillation and flutter after coronary artery bypass grafting. J Thorac Cardiovasc Surg 1990;100:338-4.
4. Chee T, Prakash N, Desser K, Benchimol A. Postoperative supraventricular arrhythmias and the role of prophylactic digoxin in cardiac surgery. Am Heart J 1982;104:974-977.
5. Davison R, Hartz R, Kaplan K, Parker M, Feiereisel P, Michaelis L. Prophylaxis of supraventricular tachyarrhythmias after coronary artery bypass surgery with oral verapamil: a randomized, double-blinded trial. Ann Thorac Surg 1985;39:336-339.
6. Pandozi C, Bianconi L, Villani M, Gentilucci G, Castro A, Altamura G, Jesi AP, Lamberti F, Ammirati F, Santini M. Elecrophysiological characteristics of the human atria after cardioversion of persistent atrial fibrillation. Circulation 1998;98:2860-2865.
7. Wiffels MCEF, Kirchhof CJHJ, Dorland R, Allessie MA. AF begets AF: a study in awake chronically instrumented goats. Circulation 1996;92:1954-1968.
8. Mathew JP, Parks R, Savino JS, Friedman AS, Koch C, Mangano DT, Browner WS. Atrial fibrillation following coronary artery bypass graft surgery: predictors, outcomes, and resource utilization. Multicenter Study of Perioperative Ischemia Research Group. J Am Med Assoc 1996 ;276:300-6.
9. Frost L, Molgaard H, Christiansen EH, Jacobsen CJ, Allermand H, Thomsen PE. Low vagal tone and supraventricular ectopic activity predict atrial fibrillation and flutter after coronary artery bypass grafting. Eur Heart J 1995;16:825-31.
10. Almassi GH, Schowalter T, Nicolosi AC, Aggarwal A, Moritz TE, Henderson WG, Tarazi R, Shroyer AL, Sethi GK, Grover FL, Hammermeister KE. Atrial fibrillation after cardiac surgery: a major morbid event?. Ann Surg 1997;226:501-513.

11. Ong JJ, Hsu PC, Lin L, Yu A, Kass RM, Peter CT, Swerdlow CD. Arrhythmias after cardioverter-defibrillator implantation: comparison of epicardial and transvenous systems. Am J Cardiol 1995;75:137-140.

12. Aranki SF, Shaw DP, Adams DH, Rizzo RJ, Couper GS, VanderVliet M, Collins JJ Jr, Cohn LH, Burstin HR. Predictors of atrial fibrillation after coronary artery surgery. Current trends and impact on hospital resources. Circulation 1996;94:390-7.

13. Hashimoto K, Ilstrup DM, Schaff HV. Influence of clinical and hemodynamic variables on risk of supraventricular tachycardia after coronary artery bypass. J Thorac Cardiovasc Surg 1991;101:56-65.

14. Stafford PJ, Kolvekar S, Cooper J, Fothergill J, Schlindwein F, deBono DP, Spyt TJ, Garratt CJ. Signal averaged P wave compared with standard electrocardiography or echocardiography for prediction of atrial fibrillation after coronary bypass grafting. Heart 1997;77:417-22.

15. Frost L, Lund B, Pilegaard H, Christiansen EH. Re-evaluation of the role of P-wave duration and morphology as predictors of atrial fibrillation and flutter after coronary artery bypass surgery. Eur Heart J 1996;17:1065-71.

16. Zaman AG, Alamgir F, Richens T, Williams R, Rothman MT, Mills PG. The role of signal averaged P wave duration and serum magnesium as a combined predictor of atrial fibrillation after elective coronary artery bypass surgery. Heart 1997;77:527-31.

17. Mooe T, Gullsby S, Rabben T, Eriksson P. Sleep-disordered breathing: a novel predictor of atrial fibrillation after coronary artery bypass surgery. Coron Art Dis 1996;7:475-8.

18. Kalman JM, Munawar m, Howes LG, Louis WJ, Buxton BF, Gutteridge G, Tonkin AM. Atrial fibrillation after coronary artery bypass grafting is associated with sympathetic activation. Ann Thorac Surg 1995;60:1709-1715.

19. Fuller JA, Adams GG, Buxton B. Atrial fibrillation after coronary artery bypass grafting: is it a disorder of the elderly? J Thorac Cardiovasc Surg 1989;97:821-825.

20. Benjamin EJ, Levy D, Vaziri SM, D'Agostino RB, Belanger AJ, Wolf PA. Independent risk factors for atrial fibrillation in a population-based cohort. The Framingham Heart Study. JAMA 1994;271:840-844.

21. Dimmer C, Jordaens L, Gorgov N, Peene I, Francois K, Van Nooten G, Clement DL. Analysis of the P wave with signal averaging to assess the risk of atrial fibrillation after coronary artery bypass surgery. Cardiol 1998;89:19-24.

22. Caretta Q, Mercanti CA, DeNardo D, Chiarotti F, Scibilia G, Reale A, Marino B. Ventricular conduction defects and atrial fibrillation after coronary artery bypass grafting. multivariate analysis of preoperative, intraoperative and postoperative variables. Eur J Cardiol 1991;12:1107-1111.

23. Steinberg JS, Zelenkofske S, Wong SC, Gelernt M, Sciacca R, Menchavez E. Value of the P-wave signal-averaged ECG for predicting atrial fibrillation after cardiac surgery. Circulation 1993;88:2618-22.

24. Creswell LL, Schuessler RB, Rosenbloom M, Cox JL. Hazards of postoperative atrial arrhythmias. Ann Thorac Surg 1993;56:539-49.

25. Frost L, Jacobsen CJ, Christiansen EH, Molgaard H, Pilegaard H, Hjortholm K, Thomsen PE. Hemodynamic predictors of atrial fibrillation or flutter after coronary artery bypass grafting. Acta Anaesth Scand 1995;39:690-7.

26. Mendes LA, Connelly GP, McKenney PA, Podrid PJ, Cupples LA, Shemin RJ, Ryan TJ, Davidoff R. Right coronary artery stenosis: an independent predictor of atrial fibrillation after coronary artery bypass surgery. J Amer Coll Cardiol 1995;25:198-202.

27. Pehkonen EJ, Mäkynen PJ, Katajo MJ, Tarkka MR. Atrial fibrillation after blood and crystalloid cardioplegia in CABG patients. Thorac Cardiovasc Surgeon 1995; 43:200-203.

28. Chew JT, Ong KK. Atrial arrhythmias post coronary bypass grafting. Singapore Med J 1993;34:430-4.

29. Akins CW. Noncardioplegic myocardial preservation for coronary revascularization. J Thorac Cardiovasc Surg 1984;88:174-181.

30. Klein M, Evans SJ, Blumberg S, Cataldo L, Bodenheimer MM. Use of p-wave triggered, p-wave signal-averaged electrocardiogram to predict atrial fibrillation after coronary artery bypass surgery. Am Heart J 1995;129:895-901.

31. Stephenson LW, MacVaugh H, Tomasello DN, Josephson ME. Propranolol for the prevention of postoperative cardiac arrhythmias: A randomized study. Ann Thorac Surg 1980;29:113-116.

32. Han J, Moe GK. Nonuniform recovery of excitability in ventricular muscle. Circ Res 1964;14:44-

60.

33. Michelucci A, Padeletti L, Fradella GA. Atrial refractoriness and spontaneous or induced atrial fibrillation. Acta Cardiol 1982;5:333-344.

34. Ali IM, Sanalla AA, Clark V. Beta-blocker effects on postoperative atrial fibrillation. Eur J Cardio-Thor Surg 1997;11:1154-7.

35. Frost L, Molgaard H, Christiansen EH, Hjortholm K, Paulsen PK, Thomsen PE. Atrial fibrillation and flutter after coronary artery bypass surgery: epidemiology, risk factors and preventive trials. Inter J Cardiol 1992;36:253-61.

36. Frost L, Molgaard H, Christiansen EH, Jacobsen CJ, Pilegaard H, Thomsen PE. Atrial ectopic activity and atrial fibrillation/flutter after coronary artery bypass surgery. A case-base study controlling for confounding from age, beta-blocker treatment, and time distance from operation. Int J Cardiol 1995;50:153-62.

37. Abel RM, Van Gelder HM, Pores IH, Liguori J, Geilchinsky I, Parsonnet V. Continued propranolol administration following coronary bypass surgery. Arch Surg 1983;118:727-731.

38. Silverman NA, Wright R, Levitsky S. Efficacy of low-dose propranolol in preventing postoperative supraventricular tachyarrhythmias. Ann Surg 1982196:194-197.

39. Salazar C, Frishman W Friedman S et al. Betablocker therapy for supraventricular tachyarrhythmias after coronary surgery: a propranolol withdrawal syndrome? Angiology 1979;30:816-819.

40. White HD, Antman GM, Glynn MA, et al. Efficacy and safety of timolol for the prevention of supraventricular tachyarrhythmias after coronary artery bypass surgery. Circulartion 1984;70:479-484.

41. Sun LS, Adams DC, Delphin E, Graham J, Meltzer E, Rose EA, Heyer EJ. Sympathetic response during cardiopulmonary bypass: mild versus moderate hypothermia. Crit Care Med 1997;25:1990-3.

42. Leier CV, Meacham JA, Schaal SF. Prolonged atrial conduction: A major predisposing factor for the development of atrial flutter. Circulation 1978;57:213-216.

43. Watson RM, Josephson ME. Atrial flutter: I. Electrophysiologic substrates and modes of initiation and termination. Am J Cardiol 1980;45:732-741.

44. Buxton AE, Josephson ME. The role of p-wave duration as a predictor of postoperative atrial arrhythmias. Chest 1981;80:68-73.

45.Guidera SA, Steinberg JS. The signal-averaged p-wave duration: a rapid and non-invasive marker of risk of atrial fibrillation. J Am Coll Cardiol 1993;21:1645-1651.

46. Ehlert FA, Gaur A, Steinberg JS. Correlation of the p-wave signal averaged electrocardiogram to intra-cardiac atrial conduction. Circulation 1996;94:I-70.

47. Hogue CWJr, Domitrovich PP, Stein PK, Despontis GD, Re L, Schuessler RB, Kleiger RE, Rottman JN. RR interval dynamics before atrial fibrillation in patients after coronary artery bypass graft surgery. Circulation 1998;98:429-434.

48. Hutchinson LA, Steinberg JS. A prospective study of atrial fibrillation after cardiac surgery: multivariate analysis using p wave signal-averaged ECG and clinical variables. Ann Noninv Elec 1996;1:133-140.

49. Gardin J, Singer D. Atrial infarction: importance, diagnosis and localization. Arch Intern Med 1981;141:1345-1348.

50. Lazar E, Goldberger J, Peled H, Sherman M, Frishman W. Atrial infarction: diagnosis and management. Am J Cardiol 1988;116:1058-1061.

51. Rechavia E, Strasberg B, Mager A et al. The incidence of atrial arrhythmias during inferior wall infarction with and without right ventricular involvement. Am Heart J 1992;124:387-391.

52. Salem BI, Chaudhry A, Haikal M, Gowda S, Campbell A, Coordes C, Leidenfrost R. Sustained supraventricular tachyarrhythmias following coronary artery bypass surgery comparing mammary versus saphenous vein grafts. Angiology 1991;42:441-6.

53. Subramanian VA, McCabe JC, Geller CM. Minimally invasive direct coronary artery bypass grafting: two-year clinical experience. Ann Thorac Surg 1997;64:1648-55.

54. Arom KV, Emery RW, Nicoloff DM, Flavin TF, Emery AM. Minimally invasive direct coronary artery bypass grafting: experimental and clinical experiences. Ann Thorac Surg 1997;63:S48-S52.

55. Tamis JE, Vloka ME, Malhotra S, Mindich BP, Steinberg JS. Atrial fibrillation is common after minimally invasive direct coronary artery bypass surgery. J Am Coll Cardiol 1998;'31:118A.

56. Michelson EL, Morganroth J, MacVaugh H. Postoperative arrhythmias after coronary artery and cardiac valvular surgery detected by long term electrocardiographic monitoring. Am Heart J 1979; 97:442-8.

57. Rouson ia, Meeran MK, Engelman RM, Breyer RH, Lemeshou S. Does the type of venous drainage or cardioplegia affect postoperative conduction and atrial arrhythmias? Circulation 1985;72:II-259-II-263.

58. Ormerod OJM, McGregor CGA, Stone DL, Wisbey C, Petch MC. Arrhythmias after coronary bypass surgery. Br Heart J 1984;51:618-621.

59. Arom KV, Emery RW, Petersen RJ, Bero JW. Evaluation of 7,000+ patients with two different routes of cardioplegia. Ann Thorac Surg 1997;63:1619-24.

60. Smith PK, Buhran WC, Levett JM, Ferguson TB Jr, Holman WL, Cox JL. Supraventricular conduction abnormalities following cardiac operations. A complication of inadequate atrial preservation. J. Thorac Cardiovasc Surg 1983;85:105-115.

61. Chen XZ, Newman M, Rosenfeldt FL. Internal cardiac cooling improves atrial preservation: electrophysiological and biochemical assessment. Ann Thorac Surg 1988;46:406-411.

62. Tchervenkov CI, Wynands JE, Symes JF, Malcolm ID, Dobell RC. Persistent atrial activity during cardioplegic arrest: A possible factor in the etiology of postoperative supraventricular tachyarrhythmias. Ann of Thorac Surg 1983;36:437-443.

63. Dewar ML, Rosengarten MD, Blundell PR, Chiu RCJ. Perioperative Holter monitoring and computer analysis of dysarrhythmias and cardiac surgery. Chest 1985;87:593-597.

64. Mullen JC, Kahn N, Weisel RD, Christakis GT, Teoh KH, Madonik MM, Mickle DAG, Ivanov J. Atrial activity during cardioplegia and postoperative arrhythmias. J Thoracic Cardiovasc Surg 1987;94:558-565.

65. Yousif H, Davies G, Oakley CM. Peri-operative supraventricular arrhythmias in coronary bypass surgery. Inter J Cardiol 1990;26:313-8.

66. Scheinman MM, Sullivan RW, Hyatt KN. Magnesium metabolism in patients undergoing cardiopulmonary bypass. Circulation 1969;39(Suppl 1):235-41.

67. Ellis RJ, Mavroudis C, Gardner C, Turley K, Ullyot D, Ebert PA. Relationship between atrioventricular arrhythmias and the concentration of K + ion in cardioplegic solution. J Thorac Cardiovasc Surg 1980;80:517-526.

68. Sharon M, Horowitz LN. Acute myocardial infarction. In Current Managemment of Arrhythmias, Horowitz LN ed. Philadelphia, B.C.Decker Inc,1991:257-64.

69. Parikka H, Toivonen L, Pellinen T, Verkkala K, Jarvinen A, Nieminen MS. The influence of intravenous magnesium sulphate on the occurrence of atrial fibrillation after coronary artery by-pass operation. Euro Heart J 1993;14:251-8.

70. Nurozler F, Tokgozoglu L, Pasaoglu I, Boke E, Ersoy U, Bozer AY. Atrial fibrillation after coronary artery bypass surgery: predictors and the role of MgSO4 replacement. J Card Surg 1996;11:421-7.

71. Fanning WJ, Thomas CS, Roach A, Tomichek R, Alford WC, Stoney WS. Prophylaxis of atrial fibrillation with magnesium sulfate after coronary atery bypass grafting . Ann Thorac Surg 1991;52:529-533.

72. Crosby LH, Pifalo WB, Woll KR, Burkholder JA. Risk factors for atrial fibrillation after coronary artery bypass grafting. AM J Cardiol 1990;66:1520-1522.

73. Page P, Plumb VJ, Okumura K, Waldo AL. A new model of atrial flutter. J Am Coll Cardiol 1986;8:872-875.

74. Kumagai K, Khrestian C, Waldo AL. Simultaneous multisite mapping studies during induced atrial fibrillation in the sterile pericarditis model. Insights into the mechanism of its maintenance. Circulation 1995;2:511-521.

75. Massie E, Valle AR. Cardiac arrhythmias complicating total pneumonectomy. Ann Intern Med 1947;26:231-239.

76. Cerney CI. The prophylaxis of cardiac arrhythmias complicating pulmonary surgery. J Thorac Surg 1957;34:105-110.

5 THE IMPACT OF ATRIAL FIBRILLATION ON HOSPITAL LENGTH OF STAY AFTER CARDIAC SURGERY

Jacqueline E. Tamis, MD and
Jonathan S. Steinberg, MD,
St. Luke's-Roosevelt Hospital Center and
Columbia University College of Physicians and
Surgeons, New York, NY

1. Introduction

The economic burden of healthcare expenditures remains a substantial concern nationwide. Physicians, third party payers and governmental agencies have begun to focus on methods to contain costs while maintaining high standards of health care delivery. During this era of widespread healthcare reform, considerable emphasis has been placed on cardiac surgery, a major contributor to gross expenditures. Approximately 500,000 cardiothoracic surgery procedures are performed each year [1] at an estimated cost of $45,000 per procedure [2]. Hospital length of stay after cardiac surgery is an important determinant of total hospital charges. The institution of critical pathways including same day admissions, early extubation, early transfer out of the intensive care unit, and early ambulation, has successfully shortened hospital length of stay after surgery without any adverse effects on morbidity or mortality [3-11]. Several reports have demonstrated a significant decrease in total hospital charges related to cardiac surgery as a result of these modifications [6-9].

Many risk assessment profiles have been performed in an attempt to identify a group of patients who are more likely to have an extended hospitalization.

This enables the health care delivery team to estimate bed allocation, and focus on individual patient recovery. The identification of these patients can also be used to advantage if attempts to modify these risks are undertaken in an effort to shorten the predicted length of stay and contain hospital costs.

Increasing age appears to be the most consistent variable contributing to prolonged post-operative length of stay [12-20]. Although length of stay in the elderly population may be influenced by the higher rate of associated comorbidities, many researchers have demonstrated that older age is independently associated with delayed discharged after cardiac surgery [13-15,18]. Patients with a history of congestive heart failure or compromised left ventricular function are also at higher risk for prolonged post-operative length of stay [5,12,13,17]. These patients are generally sicker, with more extensive coronary artery disease and/or prior myocardial infarctions. Their delayed recovery is likely related to prolonged intubation and prolonged ICU stays [18,21]. Diabetes [5,14], unstable angina [13,14,17], renal insufficiency/failure [5,15], non-CABG cardiac surgery [5,12,14], and repeat cardiac surgery [5] may also delay discharge. Reports of these patient characteristics however have not been consistent.

Atrial fibrillation, the most prevalent sustained arrhythmia seen after cardiac surgery, has been recognized as a common and potentially dangerous arrhythmia since the introduction of cardiac surgery in the 1950s [22-24]). Over the ensuing 40 years, substantial research has focused on the incidence, risk factors, treatment and prevention of this stubborn post-operative arrhythmia. With the institution of more effective medical therapy designed to treat atrial fibrillation and its associated complications, it is no longer considered a serious complication of cardiac surgery. A frequent concern of physicians treating cardiac surgery patients relates to the potential impact of atrial fibrillation on the utilization of hospital resources, particularly hospital length of stay. Several studies have demonstrated that atrial fibrillation significantly prolongs post-operative length of stay [25-32]. The purpose of this chapter is to explore the impact of atrial fibrillation on hospital length of stay after cardiac surgery.

2. Atrial Fibrillation and Length of Stay

2.1. Hospital length of stay

Approximately 25 years ago, Angelini et al [33] first described the potential relationship of atrial fibrillation to hospital length of stay after cardiac surgery. They reported on the incidence of post-operative arrhythmias in a group of 178 patients referred for cardiac surgery. Among 78 patients undergoing coronary artery bypass surgery, 7 developed atrial fibrillation. The patients who developed atrial fibrillation had a longer hospital stay than those who remained in sinus rhythm. The difference in length of stay among the 2 groups however, was small and unlikely to have been statistically significant.

Several years later in a study designed to examine the efficacy of prophylactic therapy on the prevention of atrial fibrillation, Rubin et al [29] examined 150 patients undergoing bypass surgery. Patients were excluded from enrollment if they had a left ventricular ejection fraction of less than 50%, or if they experienced an intra-operative myocardial infarction or cerebro-vascular accident. Enrolled patients were randomized to treatment with digoxin, or a combination of digoxin and propanolol, or placebo. Patients treated with digoxin and propanolol were significantly less likely to develop atrial fibrillation. Regardless of treatment assignment, the development of atrial fibrillation resulted in a longer hospital length of stay when compared with patients who remained in sinus rhythm (14.4 ± 6 days vs 12.4 ± 4 days, $p<0.02$). There were otherwise no significant differences in morbidity or mortality among the 2 groups of patients. In a recent trial by Kowey et al [30] of 157 patients randomized to digoxin or digoxin and acebutolol, the authors demonstrated nearly identical results: atrial fibrillation significantly prolonged post-operative length of stay irrespective of treatment assignment.

The small number of patients included in these analyses, and the select populations examined prohibit generalization of these results to all cardiac surgery patients. More recently, there have been several reports examining large registries of patients referred for cardiac surgery allowing one to make more appropriate estimates of the effect of atrial fibrillation on hospital length of stay [25-27]. In a prospective registry examining consecutive patients referred for cardiac surgery among 14 Veterans Administration hospitals [27], Almassi et al reported on the incidence, predictors, and outcome of post-operative atrial fibrillation. Among 3,855 patients examined, 1,141 patients (29.6%) developed atrial fibrillation. Patients who developed atrial fibrillation were hospitalized for 3 days longer than patients who remained in sinus rhythm (median stay: 10 days vs 7 days, $p<0.001$). Patients with atrial fibrillation were older and more likely to have chronic obstructive pulmonary disease, and hypertension. They were also more likely to have a complicated post-operative course including re-admission to the CCU, peri-operative MI, stroke, respiratory failure, and congestive heart failure. Since these variables might all impact on post-operative recovery, it is unclear whether atrial fibrillation was solely responsible for the delay in discharge. Similar results were reported in several other trials [25,26]. These authors also did not adjust post-operative length of stay for other potentially confounding variables.

In 2 other studies, investigators examined various pre-, intra-, and post-operative variables in order to determine which factors independently delayed discharge after heart surgery [5,13]. Lazar et al [5] demonstrated that 59% of patients with an arrhythmia had a mean post-operative length of stay over 7 days, compared with 24% of patients without an arrhythmia ($p<0.001$). Weintraub et al [13] reported similar results with 24.5% of patients with an arrhythmia and 9.2% of patients who were arrhythmia-free discharged after the tenth post-operative day ($p<0.0001$). In both of these studies, multivariate analysis demonstrated that the occurrence of a post-operative arrhythmia was an independent predictor of a prolonged post-operative length of stay. These findings however were not specific to patients with atrial fibrillation, as the definition of a post-operative arrhythmia also included bradyarrhythmias, and ventricular-tachyarrhythmias.

Montague et al [34] looked at the effect of atrial fibrillation on post-operative length of stay in 597 patients over 70 years of age referred for coronary artery bypass surgery. They demonstrated that the development of a major post-operative complication was the only independent variable predictive of a prolonged hospitalization; atrial fibrillation did not affect the hospital length of stay in this select group of patients. As this study was limited exclusively to the elderly, these findings cannot be extrapolated to the general population.

All of these earlier reports made no attempt to demonstrate an independent relationship of atrial fibrillation to hospital length of stay after cardiac surgery. We examined a prospective cohort of 216 consecutive and unselected patients referred for coronary artery bypass surgery to determine whether atrial fibrillation independently prolonged post-operative length of stay and which other variables contributed to a longer hospitalization [32]. Among 16 variables examined, the univariate predictors of a prolonged length of stay included: age ($p<0.001$), pre-operative left ventricular ejection fraction ($p<0.001$), absence of a prior smoking history ($p<0.05$), bypass limited to venous conduits ($p<0.001$), post-operative atrial fibrillation ($p<0.001$), and the occurrence of a post-operative event ($p<0.001$). length of stay for patients who developed atrial fibrillation was significantly longer than for patients who did not (15.1 ± 9.0 vs 10.0 ± 4.6 days, $p<0.001$). Even after adjusting for other significant variables, the occurrence of atrial fibrillation after bypass surgery independently prolonged length of stay: Patients who developed atrial fibrillation stayed 3.2 ± 1.7 days longer than patients who did not ($p<0.001$) (Figure 1).

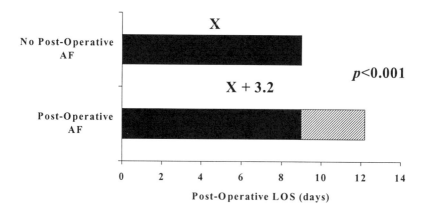

Figure 1. Relative length of stay in the presence or absence of atrial fibrillation. Patients who developed atrial fibrillation were hospitalized more than 3 days longer than patients who were free of this arrhythmia, even after accounting for differences in other baseline variables. (Adapted from Tamis et al [32]) (AF=atrial fibrillation, LOS=length of stay, x=relative length of stay for patients without atrial fibrillation).

Similar findings were later reported in a study examining a prospective cohort of 570 consecutive patients referred for coronary artery bypass surgery [28]. In this study, specific variables collected prospectively and from chart review were examined to identify the clinical predictors of post-operative atrial fibrillation. One hundred and eighty nine patients (33%) developed atrial fibrillation. The development of atrial fibrillation resulted in a prolonged post-operative length of stay (15.3 ± 28.6 days vs 9.3 ± 19.6 days, $p=0.001$). Length of stay was also affected by increasing age, gender, and the development of a significant post-operative complication. After adjusting for these variables, patients who developed atrial fibrillation were hospitalized for 4.9 additional days compared with patients who remained in sinus rhythm.

In a recent study of 2,035 consecutive patients referred for coronary artery bypass surgery, Herlitz et al [31] examined multiple pre-, intra-, and post-operative variables to determine which contributed to a post-operative length of stay over 14 days. Multivariate analysis demonstrated that the presence of a supraventricular arrhythmia significantly increased the likelihood of an extended hospitalization (RR for length of stay > 14 days for atrial fibrillation patients compared with patients free of this arrhythmia: 1.23, 95% CI 1.11-1.37, $p<0.0001$). The results reported in these recent studies have conclusively demonstrated that atrial fibrillation independently prolongs post-operative length of stay after cardiac surgery.

2.2. ICU length of stay

Patient costs incurred from the intensive care unit can be substantial; Daily charges for an intensive care unit bed are generally 2 or 3 times larger than the charges for a general medical-surgical unit and average laboratory expenses accumulated during the short stay in the intensive care unit far exceed those accrued during the remaining hospitalization [35,36]. Since intensive care unit monitoring is standard for the majority of cardiac surgery patients in the immediate post-operative period, patients requiring excessive intensive care unit care may actually interfere with the number of surgical procedures that can be performed at a given institution by preventing access to intensive care unit beds. Therefore, prolonged intensive care unit stays can significantly elevate individual patient costs, and may affect the scheduling of other elective surgical procedures.

It would be hypothesized that the occurrence of atrial fibrillation may delay transfer out of the intensive care unit due to the potential need for closer hemodynamic monitoring or infusion of potent antiarrhythmic agents. Several researchers have demonstrated that patients who developed post-operative atrial fibrillation were more likely to have a longer intensive care unit stay and had a higher incidence of readmission to the intensive care unit [25-28,37]. One study however, saw no association between post-operative atrial fibrillation and intensive care unit duration [35]. The former reports all failed to examine the temporal relationship of atrial fibrillation to intensive care unit stay. Therefore it is impossible to conclusively determine whether atrial fibrillation developed prior to, or after transfer out of the intensive care unit. Furthermore, since the independent association of atrial fibrillation and intensive care unit duration was never explored, it is difficult to conclude a causal relationship between post-operative atrial fibrillation and extended stay in the intensive care unit; Factors which are responsible for prolonged stay in the intensive care unit, including older age, compromised left ventricular function, respiratory failure and use of inotropic agents [21] are also inciting factors for the development of atrial fibrillation [25-28,38]. In the presence of these other potentially aggravating variables, one cannot be sure whether atrial fibrillation was uniquely responsible for the longer intensive care unit stay, or whether the events which resulted in prolonged intensive care unit stay also precipitated atrial fibrillation, an incidental finding.

3. Duration of Atrial Fibrillation and Length of Stay

The studies which report on the affect of atrial fibrillation on hospital length of stay have incorporated different atrial fibrillation endpoints: Some researchers defined atrial fibrillation as any sustained episode (even very short-lived) [13,25,29,30,38,39], other researchers only included clinically significant episodes of atrial fibrillation (or atrial fibrillation lasting for longer time periods) [28,31,32], and still others did not specifically define an atrial fibrillation endpoint [26,27]. One would expect that only clinically evident and prolonged durations of atrial fibrillation would effect post-operative length of stay, while short-lived or asymptomatic episodes may not have any consequence.

In a retrospective study of randomly selected patients referred for coronary artery bypass surgery (unpublished data), we examined varying durations of atrial fibrillation to determine which affected hospital length of stay. Patients were grouped according to the longest duration of atrial fibrillation recorded in the post-operative period; comparisons were made for patients with episodes of atrial fibrillation lasting for less than 6 hours with those patients who had atrial fibrillation lasting at least 24 hours. Regardless of the duration of the arrhythmia, patients who developed post-operative atrial fibrillation had a longer length of stay than patients who remained in sinus rhythm (9.5 ± 4.5 days vs 6.5 ± 2.0 days, $p<0.01$ for atrial fibrillation less than 6 hours vs. no atrial fibrillation, and 13.2 ± 6.3 days vs. 6.5 ± 2.0 days $p<0.001$ for atrial fibrillation at least 24 hours vs. no atrial fibrillation). However, there was a trend toward a longer length of stay with longer durations of atrial fibrillation ($p=0.06$ for atrial fibrillation over 24 hours compared with atrial fibrillation less than 6 hours) (Figure 2). This preliminary information is important as it implies that although all episodes of atrial fibrillation will likely impact on length of stay, prolonged episodes of atrial fibrillation are more likely to substantially delay discharge. Hence, even if atrial fibrillation develops, it's treatment and conversion to sinus rhythm remains an important option in cost containment.

4. Mechanisms for the Increased Length of Stay

Among all of the studies that have reported on the effects of atrial fibrillation on hospital length of stay, none have definitively explored the mechanisms whereby atrial fibrillation delays discharge. Some researchers have proposed that the complications occurring in association with post-operative atrial fibrillation including strokes, longer ICU stays, and higher rates of return to the ICU were responsible for the delayed discharge after bypass surgery [25-27]. However, other studies could not attribute these longer hospitalizations to such complications: Rubin et al [29] demonstrated similar morbidity for atrial fibrillation patients when compared with patients who remained in sinus rhythm while others [28,31,32] reported that even after adjustment for other potentially confounding variables including a major complication, atrial fibrillation still prolonged hospital length of stay after surgery. In these studies, the longer hospitalizations detected among patients with atrial fibrillation appeared to be independent of an increase in post-operative events and were likely a consequence of the time alloted to the evaluation and treatment of this arrhythmia.

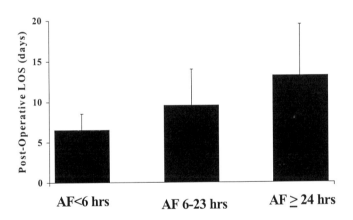

Figure 2. Post-operative length of stay (in days) for patients with no atrial fibrillation compared with patients with atrial fibrillation lasting less than 6 hours and atrial fibrillation lasting at least 24 hours. See text for detail. (AF=atrial fibrillation; hrs=hours; LOS=length of stay)

Since atrial fibrillation is frequently self-limiting, many physicians choose to observe these patients for a short time period prior to attempting cardioversion or initiating long-term anticoagulant therapy [40,41]. Even if definitive therapy is instituted early in the course of atrial fibrillation, discharge may still be delayed while attempting to achieve a therapeutic level of oral anticoagulation, or initiating pharmacologic therapy with antiarrhythmic agents. These impediments to discharge may be especially pronounced in situations where atrial fibrillation occurs later in the post-operative period when patients are already anticipating discharge.

5. Cost Implications

Additional costs incurred from post-operative atrial fibrillation are likely attributable to an increase in utilization of hospital resources as well as an increase in hospital length of stay. In a recent report [30], the authors explored the costs related to cardiac surgery for patients who developed atrial fibrillation compared with patients who remained in sinus rhythm. They found that average hospital charges for patients with atrial fibrillation were nearly 50% higher than those for patients who remained free of this arrhythmia ($74,561 vs $53,057, $p<0.05$). When hospital charges for the 2 groups were itemized, room charges accounted for over 20% of the total charges incurred during cardiac surgery and were over 50% higher for atrial fibrillation patients ($17,884 vs $10,894 $p<0.05$). Although other hospital charges were also higher for patients with atrial fibrillation, they were not significantly different than those for patients in sinus rhythm (Figure 3). These findings suggest that the most important contribution to increased costs arising from cardiac surgery for patients with atrial fibrillation result from a prolongation in hospital length of stay.

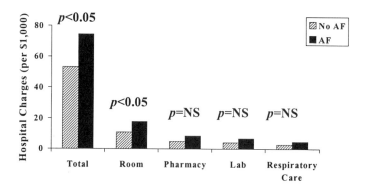

Figure 3. Hospital charges (in thousands of dollars) for cardiac surgery in the presence or absence of atrial fibrillation. Total charges and room charges were significantly higher for patients with atrial fibrillation compared with those who were arrhythmia free (Adapted from Kowey et al [30]) (AF=atrial fibrillation)

Taylor et al [35] and Mauldin et al [42] examined the effect of post-operative complications on total hospital costs related to cardiac surgery. They found that atrial fibrillation (or the presence of a major arrhythmia) was one of the most common post-operative complications. Although this complication was relatively inexpensive when compared with other more adverse events, the authors postulated that due to it's frequent occurrence, atrial fibrillation would be expected to substantially impact on total hospital charges in the health care community. Aranki et al [28] estimated that the increased length of stay attributable to atrial fibrillation resulted in an additional $10,055 to $11,500 of charges per patient. Assuming that costs for cardiac surgery nationwide are similar to those reported by Aranki et al, and if we estimate that 500,000 cardiothoracic surgery procedures are performed annually [1] and one fourth of these patients develop atrial fibrillation, then the increase in hospital stay resulting from atrial fibrillation would be expected to increase total health care charges by about **1.25 billion dollars annually**– an enormous economic burden!

6.   Methods to Improve Post-Operative Length of Stay

6.1. Prevention

One of the simplest approaches to improve length of stay after cardiac surgery may be through the prevention of post-operative atrial fibrillation. Over the past 15 years extensive therapeutic options aimed at the prevention of atrial fibrillation after cardiac surgery have been explored. Beta-adrenergic blocking agents and more recently, amiodarone therapy, appear to be the most successful method of prophylaxis [29,30,34,39,43-45]. Few investigators however have attempted to determine whether successful prevention of this arrhythmia translates into earlier discharge home.

In a study by Kowey et al. [30], 157 patients undergoing coronary artery bypass surgery were randomly assigned to treatment with digoxin and acebutolol versus digoxin alone. There was a tendency towards a lower incidence of atrial fibrillation among patients treated with acebutolol and digoxin when compared with those treated with digoxin alone, however the difference was not statistically significant. Although the authors demonstrated a longer length of stay for patients with atrial fibrillation compared with patients who were arrhythmia free, there was no significant difference in hospital length of stay between the 2 treatment groups. The lack of a significant therapeutic effect with this prophylactic regimen likely accounts for the inability of these authors to significantly improve length of stay through preventive measures.

In an article by Daoud et al [39], patients were randomized to oral amiodarone therapy administered one week before cardiac surgery or placebo. They demonstrated an improvement in the incidence of post-operative atrial fibrillation for amiodarone-treated patients when compared with placebo-treated patients. Unlike the previous study, these authors reported that treatment with this agent also resulted in a shorter length of stay (6.5 ± 2.6 days for amiodarone-treated patients vs. 7.9 ± 4.3 days for placebo-treated patients, $p=0.04$). More importantly this method of prophylaxis appeared to be cost effective with lower overall hospital charges for the treatment group compared with the placebo group ($18,375 \pm $13,863 vs. $26,491 \pm $23,837, $p=0.03$) (Figure 4).

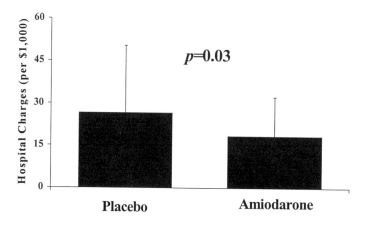

Figure 4: Hospital charges (in thousands of dollars) for patients treated with amiodarone compared with patients treated with placebo. See text for details. (Adapted from Daoud et al [39])

6.2. Early evaluation and treatment

Despite attempts at successful prophylaxis, the incidence of atrial fibrillation in many current studies remains at approximately 25% [39,30]. Among these patients, most will develop atrial fibrillation by the second or third post-operative day [39] and generally have an otherwise uncomplicated course. Although nearly all patients who develop atrial fibrillation require pharmacologic control of the ventricular response, a substantial number of patients with post-operative atrial fibrillation spontaneously convert to sinus rhythm before discharge without the need for pharmacologic or electrical cardioversion [34,38,39,41,44]. By 2 months the majority of patients with post-operative arrhythmias are in sinus rhythm irrespective of treatment [41].

Given the relative benign course of post-operative atrial fibrillation, early evaluation and intervention may likely result in earlier discharge home without any adverse effects on patient safety. We advocate that anticoagulant therapy be administered immediately in all atrial fibrillation patients (unless otherwise contraindicated) with institution of AV nodal blocking agents to control the ventricular response (preferably with beta-blockers). Patients who remain in atrial fibrillation beyond 24 hours should undergo cardioversion. In the absence of adverse events, it would be expected that most patients should be discharged within 48 hours of the development of atrial fibrillation, irrespective of whether there was successful restoration of sinus rhythm. Among those patients successfully cardioverted, antiarrhythmic drug treatment for 1-3 months after surgery can be considered. If atrial fibrillation persists at the time of discharge, oral anticoagulant therapy and rate control should be continued and titrated as an outpatient with anticipation of cardioversion at 4-6 weeks for patients who have not returned to sinus rhythm by that time.

Several authors have also advocated similar methods, with special attention to the prompt institution of therapy [28,46], aimed at early discharge home. The safety and efficacy of such an approach however is not well documented, and further investigation is needed to determine whether the prompt evaluation and treatment of patients with atrial fibrillation is reliable as well as cost effective.

7. Conclusion

Atrial fibrillation is common after cardiac surgery and results in significant prolongation of hospital length of stay independent of other potentially confounding variables. The unique effect of atrial fibrillation on hospital length of stay likely relates to the longer duration of cardiac monitoring and the time required to evaluate and treat this arrhythmia. This longer length of stay incurs substantial health care costs. Since the goal of current health care providers is to reduce health-related costs, prevention of atrial fibrillation after cardiac surgery or methods to decrease length of stay for patients who develop atrial fibrillation may significantly impact on total healthcare expenditures nationwide.

References

1. National Center for Health Statistics: Health Resources Utilization Branch –1994
2. Metropolitan Life Insurance Company-*Statistical Bulletin* 1997;78:20-28
3. Krohn BG, Kay JH, Mendez MA, Zubiate P, Kay GL. Rapid sustained recovery after cardiac operations. *J Thorac Cardiovasc Surg* 1990; 100:194-197.
4. Anderson RP, Guyton SW, Paull DL, Tidwell SL. Selection of patients for same day coronary bypass operations. *J Thorac Cardiovasc Surg* 1993; 105:444-452.
5. Lazar HL, Fitzgerald C, Gross S, Heeren T, Aldea GS, Shermin RJ. Determinants of length of stay after coronary artery bypass graft surgery. *Circulation* 1995; 92(suppl II):II-20-24.
6. Loop FD, Christiansen EK, Lester JL, Cosgrove DM, Franco I, Golding LR. A strategy for cost containment in coronary surgery. *JAMA* 1983; 250:63-66.
7. Loop FD, Higgins TL, Panda R, Pearce G, Estafanous FG. Myocardial protection during cardiac operations: decreased morbidity and lower cost with blood cardioplegia and coronary sinus perfusion. *J Thorac Cardiovasc Surg* 1992; 104:608-618.
8. Engleman RM, Rousou JA, Flack JE, et al. Fast track recovery of the coronary bypass patient. *Ann Thorac Surg* 1994; 58:1742-1746.
9. Arom KA, Emery RW, Petersen RJ and Schwartz M. Cost-Effectiveness and predictors of early extubation. *Ann Thorac Surg* 1995;60:127-132.
10. Engelman RM. Mechanisms to reduce hospital stays. *Ann of Thorac Surg* 1996;61:S26-29.
11. Cheng DCH, Karski J, Peniston C, Asokumar B, Raveendran G, et al. Morbidity outcome in early versus conventional tracheal extubation after coronary artery bypass grafting: A prospective randomized controlled trial. *J Thorac Cardiovasc Surg* 1996;112:755-764.
12. Tu JV, Jaglal SB, Naylor CD, the Steering Committee of the Provincial Adult Cardiac Care Network of Ontrario. Multicenter validation of a risk index for mortality, intensive care unit stay, and overall hospital length of stay after cardiac surgery. *Circulation* 1995; 91:677-684.
13. Weintraub WS, Jones EL, Craver J, Guyton R, Cohen C. Determinants of prolonged length of hospital stay after coronary bypass surgery. *Circulation* 1989; 80:276-284.
14. Katz NM, Ahmed SW, Clark BK, Wallace RB. Predictors of length of hospitalization after cardiac surgery. *Ann Thorac Surg* 1988; 45:656-660.

15. Lahey SJ, Borlase BC, Lavin PT, Levitsky S. Preoperative risk factors that predict hospital length of stay in coronary artery bypass patients >60 years old. *Circulation* 1992; 86(suppl II):II-181-185.

16. Katz NM, Hannan RL, Hopkins RA, Wallace RA. Cardiac operations in patients aged 70 years and over: Mortality, length of stay, and hospital charge. *Ann Thorac Surg* 1995; 60:96-101.

17. Lazar HL, Wilcox K, McCormick JR, Roberts AJ. Determinants of discharge following coronary artery bypass graft surgery. *CHEST* 1987; 92:800-803.

18. Mounsey JP, Griffith MJ, Heaviside DW, Brown AH, Reid DS. Determinants of length of stay in intensive care and in hospital after coronary artery surgery. *Br Heart J* 1995; 73:92-98.

19. Peigh PS, Swartz MT, Vaca KJ, Lohman DP, Naunheim KS. Effect of advancing age on cost and outcome of coronary artery bypass grafting. *Ann Thorac Surg* 1994; 58:1362-1367.

20. Hochberg MS, Levine FH, Daggett WM, Akins CW, Austen WG, Buckley MJ. Isolated coronary artery bypass grafting in patients seventy years of age and older. Early and late results. *J Thorac Cardiovasc Surg* 1982; 84:219-223.

21. Tu JV, Mazer D, Levinton C, Armstrong PW, and Naylor D. A predictive index for length of stay in the intensive care unit following cardiac surgery. *Can Med Assoc J* 1994;151:177-185.

22. Rogers W, Wroblewski F, LaDue JS. Supraventicular tachycardia complicating surgical procedures. *Circulation* 1955;12:192-

23. Gross H, Kepes ER, Young D, et al. Electrocardiograhic changes during mitral commissurotomy. *Am Heart J* 1957;54:863-

24. Sasaki R, Theilen EO, Jauary LE et al. Cardiac arrhythmias associated with the repair of atrial and ventricular septal defects. *Circulation* 1958;18:909-

25. Creswell LL, Schuessler RB, Rosenbloom M, Cox JL. Hazards of postoperative atrial arrhythmias. *Ann Thorac Surg* 1993; 56:539-549.

26. Mathew JP, Parks R, Savino JS, et al. Atrial fibrillation following coronary artery bypass graft surgery; predictors, outcomes and resource utilization. *JAMA* 1992; 276:300-306.

27. Almassi GH, Schowalter T, Nicolosi AC, Aggarwal A, Moritz TE, et al. Atrial fibrillation after cardiac surgery. A major morbid event? *Ann of Surg* 1997;226:501-513.

28. Aranki SF, Shaw DP, Adams DH, Rizzo RJ, Couper GS, VanderVliet M, Collins JJ, Cohn LH, Burstin HR. Predictors of atrial fibrillation after coronary artery surgery. Current trends and impact on hospital resources. *Circulation* 1996;94:390-397.

29. Rubin DA, Nieminski KE, Reed GE, Herman MV. Predictors, prevention, and long term prognosis of atrial fibrillation after coronary artery bypass graft operations. *J Thorac Cardiovasc Surg* 1987, 94:331-335.

30. Kowey PR, Dalessandro DA, Herbertson R, Briggs B, Wertan MAC et al. Effectiveness of digitalis with or without acebutolol in preventing atrial arrhythmias after coronary artery bypass surgery. *Am J Cardiol* 1997;70:1114-1117.

31. Herlitz J, Brandrup G, Emanuelsson H, Haglid M, Karlsson T, et al. Determinants of time to discharge following coronary artery bypass grafting. *Eur J Cardio-thorac Sur* 1997;11:533-538.

32. Tamis JE, Steinberg JS. Atrial Fibrillation is the only modifiable factor that lengthens hospital stay after coronary artery bypass surgery. *PACE* 1996;19:225.

33. Angelini P, Feldman MI, Lufschanowski R, Leachman RD. Cardiac arrhythmias during and after heart surgery: Diagnosis and management. *Prog in Cardiovasc Dis* 1974; 16:469-495.

34. Matangi MF, Neutze JM, Graham KJ, Hill DG, Kerr AR, et al. Arrhythmia prophylaxis after aortocoronary bypass. The effect of minidose propanolol. *J Thorac Cardiovasc Surg* 1985;89:439-443.

35. Taylor GJ, Mikell FL, Moses HW, Dove JT, Katholi RE, et al. Determinants of hospital charges for coronary artery bypass surgery: The economic consequences of post-operative complications. *Am J Cardiol* 1990;65:309-313.

36. Zenati M, Comit TM, Saul M, Gorcsan J, Katz WE, et al. Resource utilization for minimally invasive direct and standard coronary artery bypass grafting. *Ann Thorac Surg* 1997;63:S84-87.

37. Lowe JE, Hendry PJ, Hendrickson SC, and Wells R. Intraoperative indentification of cardiac patients at risk to develop postoperative atrial fibrillation. *Ann of Surg* 1991;213:388-391.

38. Hashimoto K, Ilstrup DM, and Schaff HV. Influence of clinical and hemodynamic variables on risk of supraventricular tachycardia after coronary artery bypass surgery. *J Thorac Cardiovasc Surg* 1991;101:56-65.

39. Daoud EG, Strickberger AS, Man C, Goyal R, Deeb GM, et al. Preoperative amiodarone as prophylaxis against atrial fibrillation after heart surgery. *N Engl J Med* 1997;337:1785-1791.

40. Waldo AL, Henthorn RW, Epstein AE, Plumb VJ,. Diagnosis and treatment of arrhythmias during and following cardiac surgery. *Med Clin North Am* 1984;68:1153-1170.

41. Meijer A, Wellens HJJ. Tachyarrhythmias after cardiac surgery: A practical approach toward prevention and treatment. *ACC Current J Review* 1995;53-55.

42. Mauldin PD, Weintraub WS, and Becker ER. Predicting hospital costs for first time coronary artery bypass grafting from preoperative and postoperative variables. *Am J Cardiol* 1994;74:772-775.

43. Daudon P, Corcos T, Gandjbakhch I, Levasseur JP, Cabrol A, et al. Prevention of atrial fibrillation or flutter by acebutolol after coronary artery bypass surgery. *Am J Cardiol* 1986;58:933-936.

44. Mohr R, Smolinsky A, Goor DA. Prevention of supraventricular tachyarrhythmias with low-dose propranolol after coronary bypass. *J Thorac Cardiovasc Surg* 1981; 81:840-845.

45. Kowey PR, Taylor JE, Rials SJ, and Marinchak RA. Meta-analysis of the effectiveness of prophylactic drug therapy in preventing supraventricular arrhythmia early after coronary artery bypass grafting. *Am J Cardiol* 1992;69:963-965.

46. Ommen SR, Odell JA, and Stanton MS. Atrial arrhythmias after cardiothoracic surgery. *N Engl J Med* 1997;336:1429-1434.

6 PROPHYLACTIC VALUE OF BETA BLOCKERS

Javier E. Sanchez, MD and
Andrew E. Epstein, MD,
University of Alabama at Birmingham, AL

1. Introduction

The roles and safety of beta blockade following cardiac surgery have been controversial for three decades. In the 1960's and early 1970's it was feared that perioperative use of beta blockers would cause significant myocardial depression by either their direct antiadrenergic effects or the potentiation of the myocardial depressant effects of general anesthetics. Many recommended that beta blockers be discontinued from 48 hours [1,2] to as early as 2 weeks before surgery [3]. This practice was challenged after reports of worsening angina, myocardial infarction, ventricular tachycardia, and sudden death following the abrupt cessation of beta blockers in patients treated chronically with propranolol [4,5] as well as an increased incidence of perioperative complications in patients in whom beta blockers were discontinued preoperatively [6]. By the late 1970's the safety for continued beta blockade before and after cardiac surgery was demonstrated [7,8], and this strategy was tested for the prevention of postoperative complications, most often supraventricular arrhythmias. Herein we review the clinical trials testing various beta-adrenergic antagonists after cardiac surgery for the prevention of postoperative atrial fibrillation (Table 1) and offer recommendations for treatment.

2. Clinical Trials of Propranolol

Oka et al. reported the effects of propranolol withdrawal in patients with stable angina referred for bypass surgery [9]. Fifty four consecutive patients treated with propranolol chronically and scheduled for elective surgery were randomized to three different strategies: abrupt discontinuation of therapy 48 hours before surgery, discontinuation 10 hours before surgery, or continuation of beta blockade until the day of surgery followed by low dose intravenous propranolol for 36 to 48 hours postoperatively. These three groups were compared also to 17 patients who did not receive propranolol either prior to or after surgery. The highest incidence of supraventricular arrhythmias was observed in the groups randomized to discontinuation of propranolol 48 or 10 hours before surgery when compared to the group receiving pre- and postoperative propranolol. The authors also noted a marked increase in the rate-pressure product during intubation and postoperative periods in the patients for whom the beta blocker was discontinued before surgery. The authors speculated that both findings were due to propranolol withdrawal following a hyperadrenergic response to stress.

In 1980 Stephenson et al. reported the efficacy of propranolol to prevent postoperative cardiac arrhythmias in patients undergoing coronary artery bypass surgery [10]. Two hundred twenty three patients were randomized to receive oral propranolol 10 mg every 6 hours after transfer from the surgical intensive care unit, or to usual care without beta blocker administration. Approximately 70% of patients in both groups had received beta blockers at least 4 days prior to surgery. The incidence of all cardiac arrhythmias was significantly reduced in the group receiving postoperative propranolol (23% versus 10%, p<0.05). Specifically, the incidence of atrial fibrillation and flutter was decreased from 18% in the control group to 8% in the treatment group. The possible role of beta blocker withdrawal was not investigated, but the authors concluded that the routine use of postoperative low dose oral propranolol in hemodynamically stable patients was effective in the prevention of postoperative cardiac arrhythmias.

Mohr et al. reported another series regarding the use of propranolol for the prevention of supraventricular arrhythmias following coronary artery bypass surgery [11]. Eighty five patients receiving long-term therapy before the surgery were randomized to continued beta blockade (5 mg for normotensive patients and 10 mg for hypertensive patients via nasogastric tube every 6 hours starting 6 hours postoperatively), or to no postoperative beta blocker use. Another 18 patients who had not received beta blockers preoperatively were given the same regimen of postoperative propranolol. The incidence of supraventricular arrhythmia was significantly reduced in the group that received pre- and low dose postoperative propranolol (5%) when compared to both the group that received no propranolol (40% incidence supraventricular arrhythythmias, p<0.001), and the group that received propranolol post- but –not preoperatively (27.7% incidence of supraventricular arrhythmias, p<0.01). Twenty five of the 26 supraventricular arrhythmias documented in this study were atrial fibrillation or atrial flutter. The authors noted that the postoperative low-dose propranolol was not by itself an effective prophylactic strategy as most of the benefit was seen in patients whom had received not only postoperative propranolol but also long term preoperative beta blocker therapy. It was the impression of the authors that patients not receiving preoperative beta blocker therapy did not benefit as much from those who received postoperative propranolol because by the time they had received enough drug to achieve significant beta blockade most arrhythmias had already occurred. On the other hand, those patients receiving beta blockers before surgery and given early postoperative propranolol were more effectively protected in the postoperative period. These results supported the hypothesis that hypersensitivity to postoperative adrenergic stimulation after propranolol withdrawal was a major cause of supraventricular arrhythmias. Of note, this study included patients with low left ventricular ejection fractions, left ventricular aneurysms, a history of congestive heart failure and even some patients that required norepinephrine during or after weaning from bypass, demonstrating the safety of low dose propranolol in patients traditionally felt to be poor candidates for beta blockade.

In 1982 Silverman et al. further studied the efficacy of low dose propranolol to prevent atrial fibrillation and flutter in patients who had received long-term beta blocker therapy before coronary artery bypass surgery [12]. One

Table 1. Effect of beta blockers on the incidence of atrial arrhythmias following cardiac surgery

Reference	# patients	Drug	Incidence of supraventricular arrhythmias according to treatment group (%)		
			Control	beta blocker	p value
Stephenson[10]	223	Propranolol	17.8	8.0	<0.05
Mohr[11]	105	Propranolol	39.6	5.4	<0.001
Silverman[12]	100	Propranolol	28.0	6.0	<0.01
Abel[13]	100	Propranolol	36.0	14.6	<0.05
Ivey[14]	116	Propranolol	16.1	13.2	NS
Hammond[15]	50	Propranolol	46.2	20.8	0.06
Matangi[16]	164	Propranolol	23.2	9.8	0.02
Rubin[20]	77	Propranolol	37.5	16.2	<0.03
Martinussen[17]	75	Propranolol	14.3	12.5	NS
Shafei[18]	343	Propranolol	10.8	10.4	NS
Ormerod[19]	90	Propranolol	27.3	14.8	NS
Roffman[21]	225	Propranolol and digoxin	28.2	2.2	<0.005
Mills[22]	179	Propranolol and digoxin	30.0	3.4	<0.001
White[24]	41	Timolol	100	100	NS[a]
Vecht[25]	132	Timolol	19.7	7.5	<0.05
Daudon[26]	100	Acebutolol	40.0[c]	0[c]	<0.001
Materne[27]	71	Acebutolol	33.3	3.3	<0.001
Janssen[31]	89[b]	Metoprolol[b]	36.0	15.3	<0.05
Khuri[28]	148	Nadolol	41.9	9.0	<0.001
Lamb[29]	60	Atenolol	36.7	3.3	0.001
Matangi[30]	70	Atenolol	31.4[d]	8.6[d]	<0.05

a: The total number of episodes of atrial fibrillation in the timolol and placebo groups were 5 and 291 (p<0.05) respectively.
b: Excluding group of patients treated with sotalol.
c: Incidence of atrial fibrillation or flutter.
d: Incidence of arrhythmias requiring treatment.

hundred patients were randomized to either reinstitution of propranolol 10 mg enterally every 6 hours the day after surgery or to no propranolol therapy. The incidence of postoperative atrial flutter or fibrillation was reduced from 28% in the no-treatment group (8 patients developed atrial fibrillation and 6 patients developed atrial flutter) to 6% in the group receiving early re-administration of propranolol (3 cases of atrial fibrillation, no atrial flutter, p<0.01). In this study patients with stable angina had their preoperative dose of propranolol tapered to 40 mg every 6 hours by the day before surgery or, if receiving a lower dose, continued on their home regimen. Patients with unstable angina or significant left main coronary artery disease had their usual regimen continued without change. With the above precautions more than 50% of patients with some traditional relative contraindications to beta blocker therapy (transient need for inotropic support, need for urgent revascularization, and depressed left ventricular ejection fraction) were included without significant postoperative complications.

Abel et al. tried a more aggressive strategy for the prevention of arrhythmias in patients receiving chronic beta blocker therapy undergoing coronary artery bypass surgery [13]. One hundred patients were randomized to discontinuation of preoperative beta blockade with postoperative reinstitution only if indicated for clinically important arrhythmias or hypertension, or to receive intra- and postoperative propranolol. The intraoperative regimen provided 1 mg of propranolol intravenously at the induction of anesthesia followed by another milligram at the onset of cardiopulmonary bypass. This was followed by 2 mg intravenously every 4 hours until oral administration was possible, at which time 10 mg every 6 hours for 24 hours were given, followed by 20 mg every 6 hours until the day before discharge when the dose was tapered to 10 mg every 6 hours after which the drug was discontinued. This protocol reduced the incidence of atrial fibrillation from 36% in the no-treatment group to 14.6% in the propranolol-treated group (p<0.05). In this study all patients in the treatment arm received intraoperative propranolol, but 9, including 4 who developed intraoperative or early postoperative hypotension or bradycardia requiring pacing, were excluded from further treatment with propranolol and were not included in the results. Although the study was not blinded, it is interesting that 52% of the patients randomized to no propranolol required beta blocker therapy after the surgery for usual indications. Also, the treatment group required more inotropic support during the first 24 hours postoperatively than did the group not receiving beta blockade. The authors concluded, however, that the continuation of beta blockade was safe and effective therapy to reduce the incidence of postoperative atrial arrhythmias.

Ivey et al. further studied the usefulness of propranolol for the prevention of supraventricular arrhythmias after coronary revascularization in patients receiving long term preoperative beta blockade [14]. They randomized 116 patients who were tolerating at least 80 mg of propranolol /day, had left ventricular ejection fractions greater than 0.40, and no history of atrial arrhythmias to receive either 20 mg of propranolol by mouth or placebo every 6 hours starting within 24 hours postoperatively. Patients were excluded if digoxin, quinidine or procainamide were being prescribed. The authors found that the treatment was well tolerated but that it only reduced the incidence of supraventricular arrhythmias from 16.1% in the control group to 13.2% in the treatment group. This study was the first of only a few trials in which the benefit of beta blockade did not reach statistical significance (see Table 1).

The above report was cited as one of the reasons for studying the effect of higher doses of perioperative beta blockade on the incidence of atrial arrhythmias by Hammond et al. [15]. Fifty patients with stable angina and no congestive heart failure were randomized in a double blind, placebo-controlled fashion to receive propranolol 60 mg or placebo every 6 hours starting 24 to 48 hours before the operation and the same regimen upon arrival to the intensive care unit after the operation. Forty four percent of all patients had received beta blockers long term before randomization. These patients had their beta blocker weaned over a 24 to 48 hour period after the study drug had been started. The study drug was given orally until the surgery and via a nasogastric tube immediately upon arrival to the intensive care unit after the operation. The overall incidence of arrhythmias was decreased from 58% in the control group to 29% in the treatment group, while the proportion of patients having supraventricular arrhythmias postoperatively was decreased from 46% to 21% respectively. Another salutary effect of propranolol observed in this study was a decrease in postoperative myocardial oxygen consumption as measured by the rate-pressure product. This benefit was achieved due to a decrease in the number of episodes of postoperative hypertension. The authors noted that no patient with a propranolol level greater than 75 ng/ml had arrhythmias, and that this level was not consistently achieved with an oral regimen, possibly secondary to the variation in propranolol absorption and metabolism in the different patients. The propranolol dosing regimen was well tolerated in this study and the authors recommended it for routine use in similar patient populations.

Matangi et al. also studied the effects of low dose propranolol in the incidence of postoperative atrial fibrillation in patients receiving long-term beta blockade [16]. Of 244 consecutive patients, 164 were randomized to receive either 5 mg of propranolol enterally every 6 hours starting an average of 10 hours after the operation or to serve as controls. Exclusion criteria included a left ventricular ejection fraction of less than 0.36, no preoperative use of beta blockers, congestive heart failure, postoperative atrioventricular block or the need for inotropic support. The incidence of postoperative supraventricular tachycardia, defined as either atrial fibrillation, atrial flutter and ectopic atrial tachycardia, that required antiarrhythmic therapy was reduced from 23% in the control group to 9.8% in the treatment group (p<0.02). The incidence of atrial fibrillation alone was reduced by 50%, from 14.6% in the control group to 7.3% in the treatment group. The authors also noted a significant decrease in the number of ventricular arrhythmias, a finding consistent with other studies [14]. Thus, early reinstitution of beta blockade in patients who had received preoperative beta blockade and who did not develop a contraindication postoperatively was recommended.

In 1988 two groups of investigators reported the lack of benefit of prophylactic low dose propranolol to prevent supraventricular arrhythmias following coronary bypass surgery. Martinussen et al. prospectively randomized 75 patients to receive placebo or propranolol 10 mg 4 times a day starting in the day of the surgery [17]. Supraventricular tachycardia occurred in 14.3% of the placebo treated patients versus 12.5 % in those receiving propranolol. Although there was a trend favoring the use of beta blockers, the difference was not statistically significant. In this study the occurrence of postoperative atrial arrhythmias was unrelated to preoperative beta blocker use. Similarly, Shafei et al. [18] found no significant reduction in the incidence of supraventricular arrhythmias when low dose propranolol (10 mg 3 times a day) was administered prophylactically after coronary bypass surgery. Their study included 343 consecutive patients of whom the first half did not receive prophylactic beta blockade. The incidence of supraventricular tachycardias was 10.8% in the control group versus 10.4% in the treatment group. A not statistically significant trend towards greater efficacy was observed in patients who had received long-term beta blockade preoperatively (9.9% in those who continued to receive propranolol versus 13.8% in those who did not receive propranolol postoperatively). The authors of both studies recognized the possibility of a beneficial effect of postoperative propranolol but concluded that therapy with low dose propranolol was only marginally beneficial.

Different groups have tested the relative benefits of postoperative propranolol, digoxin and placebo in the prevention of postoperative atrial fibrillation with similar results [19,20]. Rubin et al. randomized 150 patients to receive propranolol 20 mg every 6 hours starting on postoperative day 1, digoxin 0.50 mg intravenously on the day of surgery followed by 0.25 mg orally every day thereafter, or placebo [20]. Patients were excluded if there was a history of atrial fibrillation or if the left ventricular ejection fraction was less than 0.50. Digoxin was not effective in reducing the incidence of atrial fibrillation when compared to placebo (37.5% versus 32.6%, respectively). On the other hand, only 16.2% of patients receiving propranolol developed the arrhythmia (p<0.03). In this study about 30% of all patients had been taking beta blockers preoperatively and their use did not correlate with the incidence of postoperative atrial fibrillation. It is interesting that there was no increased incidence of stroke, angina, myocardial infarction, or death in the patients who suffered postoperative atrial fibrillation, even after 27 months of follow up. The authors did show a statistically significant prolongation of the hospital stay by an average of 2 days in those patients that developed atrial fibrillation. They concluded that postoperative atrial fibrillation was a "benign epiphenomenon" not necessarily requiring prophylaxis, but that its incidence could be decreased by the routine use of propranolol in patients with normal left ventricular function. Since these patients all had preserved left ventricular function, it may be expected that the benefit of perioperative beta blockade may be less than a higher risk population.

Finally, the strategy of using propranolol in conjunction with digoxin for the prevention of atrial arrhythmias after cardiac surgery has also been tested. Roffman et al. randomized 225 patients to receive digoxin alone, digoxin and propranolol, or no prophylactic medication after coronary bypass surgery [21]. The incidence of supraventricular arrhythmias was similar in the patients receiving digoxin or no prophylactic treatment (28.9% and 28.2% respectively), but was significantly decreased in the group receiving propranolol in addition to digoxin (2.2%, p<0.005). In a similar fashion, Mills et al. randomized 179 consecutive patients to receive digoxin and propranolol together or no prophylactic drug therapy after bypass surgery [22]. The patients receiving prophylactic therapy received 10 mg of propranolol enterally every 6 hours starting 6 hours after surgery and digoxin 0.25 mg intravenously every 6 hours for the first postoperative day, followed by 0.25 mg orally daily. The control group did not receive postoperative propranolol or digoxin unless clinically indicated. The incidence of atrial fibrillation or flutter was decreased from 30% in the control group to 3.4% in the treatment group (p<0.001). Most of the patients (79%) in the control group had been taking beta blockers in the preoperative period and there was a trend towards an increased incidence of arrhythmias in those patients (35% versus 26%), but this difference was not statistically significant. The authors recommended both propranolol and digoxin for the prevention of arrhythmias following coronary bypass surgery.

3. Clinical Trials of Beta Blockers Other than Propranolol

Beta adrenergic antagonists other than propranolol have also been used to prevent postoperative atrial fibrillation. Timolol, atenolol acebutolol, metoprolol, and nadolol offer the advantage of decreasing the incidence of non-cardiac side effects such as bronchospasm (possibly increasing the number of patients who could be offered the therapy) or of having longer half-lives facilitating their administration [23]. The use of antiarrhythmic agents that also posses beta blocking properties, like sotalol and amiodarone, is discussed elsewhere in this book.

White et al. randomized 41 patients undergoing coronary bypass surgery to receive timolol 0.5 mg or placebo intravenously twice a day starting within 6 hours of surgery [24]. After resuming oral intake patients continued to receive timolol 10 mg or placebo twice a day. The authors monitored the incidence of supraventricular arrhythmias with 24 hour cassette recorders. This increased surveillance together with the inclusion of well tolerated short-lived arrhythmias led to the detection of supraventricular arrhythmias in all of the patients in the study. The number of episodes of atrial fibrillation or flutter were reduced from 291 in the placebo group to 5 in the timolol group (p<0.05). Even though most of this events were of questionable clinical significance (only 4 patients required treatment in the placebo group and only 1 patient was treated in the timolol group), the authors concluded that timolol was effective for preventing postoperative atrial arrhythmias. No significant morbidity was associated with the use timolol in this group of patients with left ventricular ejection fractions greater than 40%.

Timolol was also studied by Vecht et al. [25]. One hundred twenty three patients undergoing coronary artery bypass surgery were randomized to receive oral timolol (5 mg every 12 hours for 1 day, followed by 10 mg twice day) or placebo starting 24 hours after surgery. The total number of supraventricular arrhythmias, including atrial tachycardias was significantly decreased, but the incidence of atrial fibrillation was similar in both groups. Interestingly, there was an increased incidence of atrial arrhythmias in the patients who had been receiving chronic preoperative beta blockade, but the finding did not achieve statistical significance. The authors also noted no significant decrease in the heart rate of the timolol treated patients until after the third postoperative day, suggesting that effective beta blockade may not obtained until after 72 hours following surgery. Because a significant proportion of the arrhythmias occurred during within 3 days of surgery the authors proposed the early use of intravenous timolol in the postoperative period to achieve early therapeutic drug levels.

Acebutolol, a cardioselective beta blocker has also been tested for the prevention of atrial fibrillation or flutter after bypass surgery. Daudon et al. studied 100 consecutive patients scheduled for coronary bypass surgery [26]. Patients were randomized to receive acebutolol in increasing oral doses (titrated to maintain a heart rate between 50 and 90 beats per minute) starting 36 hours after the surgery or to serve as controls. Patients were excluded for traditional contraindications to beta blockade including asthma, chronic lung disease, diabetes and significant left ventricular dysfunction. The patients in the control group that had received preoperative beta blocker therapy as part of their medical regimen experienced an increased incidence of atrial arrhythmias (46% in patients with preoperative beta blockade versus 18% in patients that had not received preoperative beta blockers), lending support to the beta blocker withdrawal hypothesis. Therapy with acebutolol was effective, reducing the incidence of atrial fibrillation from 34% in the control group to 0% in the acebutolol treated patients. The number of events in this study was small, but the results were encouraging and the authors advocated the use of beta blockers after coronary surgery for the prevention of atrial fibrillation or flutter. Similarly, acebutolol was found effective by Materne et al. in reducing the incidence of atrial fibrillation, flutter or ectopic atrial tachycardia after coronary bypass surgery [27]. In their study, 71 patients were randomized to receive either acebutolol or no routine beta blocker after surgery. The incidence of supraventricular arrhythmias was decreased from 33% in the control group to 3% in the treatment group (p<0.001). This study also documented hemodynamic variables like pulmonary wedge pressure, mean arterial pressure, and cardiac index to be similar in patients from both groups at various intervals before and after the surgery, adding more weight to the body of evidence supporting the safety of postoperative antiadrenergic therapy in patients that are stable after the operation.

Nadolol, a non selective, long-acting beta blocker was studied by Khuri et al. [28]. This agent was chosen for the practical advantage of allowing once-a-day treatment. In a double blinded fashion, 148 patients were randomized to receive nadolol (a dose equivalent to the preoperative beta blocking dose or an increasing dose of nadolol until achieving a heart rate < 75 beats per minute if no beta blocker was used before the surgery) or placebo in a similar manner. Eighty-nine percent of the patients in this study had received beta blockers preoperatively. The number of arrhythmias that required intervention was significantly reduced in the treatment group. The incidence of atrial fibrillation and flutter was also reduced (from 22% to 12%), but this reduction was not statistically significant. The drug was well tolerated and the authors recommended the routine use of postoperative nadolol at least in patients who had benefited from beta blockers before the operation.

The prophylactic use of atenolol has also been shown effective for the prevention of atrial fibrillation after elective coronary revascularization. Lamb et al. randomized 60 patients, 50% of whom were receiving preoperative beta blockers, to receive atenolol 50 mg daily starting 72 hours before the surgery or placebo [29]. Beta blockers, if used before the operation, were discontinued 72 hours before surgery in the atenolol group or continued until the day of the operation in the control group. Atenolol proved to be effective in decreasing the incidence of atrial fibrillation from 33% in the control to 3% in the treated patients. Similarly, Matangi et al. studied 70 patients undergoing elective coronary bypass surgery. Patients were randomized to placebo or atenolol early after the surgery. The authors reported a reduction in the episodes of atrial arrhythmias requiring treatment from 31.4% in the placebo group to 8.9% in the atenolol group (p<0.05). The authors of both of the above studies concluded that atenolol is a practical and effective therapy for the prevention of atrial arrhythmias following coronary artery bypass surgery. They also suggested that in view of its cardioselective properties, atenolol could be used to expand the number of patients eligible for postoperative beta blockade.

Metoprolol has also been studied for the prevention of supraventricular tachycardias following cardiac surgery. Janssen et al. reported a significant reduction in the episodes of supraventricular arrhythmias (mostly atrial fibrillation) when comparing early postoperative use of metoprolol versus therapy with no beta blocking agent in patients undergoing coronary revascularization [31]. The incidence of arrhythmias was decreased from 36% in the control group to 15.3% in the metoprolol group (p<0.05). This study included a group treated with sotalol with favorable results. The authors concluded that the postoperative use of beta blocking agents was effective in the prophylaxis of atrial arrhythmias after bypass surgery.

4. Meta-analyses

As can be appreciated from the above review, there has been a great variety in the design, number of patients enrolled, and beta blocking agents used for the prevention of atrial fibrillation following coronary artery bypass surgery. The studies have uniformly demonstrated that, when used carefully, beta blockers are safe in the postoperative period. Most trials have also showed a reduction in the number of episodes of atrial fibrillation. This impression is reinforced by the results of 2 recent meta-analysis. Kowey et al. examined the effectiveness of drug therapy for preventing supraventricular arrhythmias early after coronary bypass surgery [32]. The English literature was searched for reports on the effectiveness of beta blockers and digoxin. The studies included incorporated a placebo-control group, provided an exact description of the treatment regimen and method for detection of arrhythmias, and did not permit the use of other antiarrhythmic agents. Nine trials of beta blocking drugs were found that met their inclusion criteria, including two trials in which beta blockers were used in conjunction with digoxin. The seven trials in which beta blockers were compared to placebo included 1,418 patients. The incidence of supraventricular tachycardias was significantly less in the beta blocker (20.2%) than in the placebo group (9.8%, p<0.001). The two trials testing beta blockers in addition to digoxin versus placebo included 292 patients. The incidence of supraventricular tachycardias was 29.4% in the control subjects versus 2.2% in the treatment group (p<0.001). Of interest, five trials of digoxin versus placebo were found that met the inclusion criteria. In their analysis digoxin was of no significant benefit. The authors concluded that beta blockade is effective in the prevention of postoperative supraventricular tachycardias. They also suggested that perhaps in the presence of effective beta blockade the vagomimetic effects of digoxin are not overridden by the postoperative increase in adrenergic tone, thus enabling the drugs to work synergistically.

Andrews et al. also investigated the effectiveness of prophylactic therapy after coronary artery bypass surgery [33]. The authors performed a meta-analysis of trials using digoxin, verapamil, or beta blockers for the prevention of supraventricular arrhythmias after coronary bypass surgery. Only randomized, controlled trials of oral therapy were included. Trials in which either the study drug

104

was used intravenously, other antiarrhythmic therapy was allowed, or the period of monitoring was less than 3 days were excluded. Nineteen studies of beta blocking agents were found to meet their inclusion criteria including a trial using sotalol. In 13 of the 19 trials found, a significant benefit of beta blockade therapy was reported, and no trial documented a detrimental effect. Neither digoxin nor verapamil were found to reduce the likelihood of supraventricular arrhythmias while the prophylactic use of beta blockers markedly decreased the likelihood of postoperative arrhythmias (OR = 0.28, CI = 0.21- 0.36). Moreover, the benefit of beta blockade was seen in patients receiving both low dose and high dose propranolol as well as in patients treated with other beta blocking agents. The authors recommended the routine use of beta blockers as a prophylactic measure against supraventricular arrhythmias in patients undergoing coronary artery bypass surgery that do not have a clinical contraindication for the use of such agents.

Table 2. Meta-analyses of beta blockers following cardiac surgery

Study	No. of trials	No. of patients	Incidence of SVA[a] according to treatment group		p value
			Control (%)	beta blocker(%)	
Andrews	18	1,549	34.0	8.7	<0.0001
Kowey	7[b]	1,418	20.2	9.8	<0.001

a: Supraventricular arrhythmia
b: Trials using digoxin and beta blockers together are not included in the table.

5. Recommendations for Therapy Following Bypass Surgery

As can be appreciated from the above review, the use of beta blockers in the perioperative period has evolved from being considered detrimental to being regarded as safe and beneficial for reducing perioperative complications, most notably postoperative supraventricular arrhythmias. It is well recognized that most patients with coronary artery disease tolerate and benefit from chronic beta blocker therapy, a fact reflected by the significant number of patients receiving beta blockers before the operation in all the trials reviewed. Furthermore, it must be kept in mind that many patients undergoing bypass surgery will have suffered a recent myocardial infarction, and continued beta blockade is indicated irrespective of cardiac surgery [34]. A good argument can be made for their use simply because surgery does not "cure" coronary artery disease, and the myocardial substrate for both atrial and ventricular arrhythmias persists. The early administration of beta blockers after the operation adds to the already well recognized benefits of chronic beta blockade a reduction in the incidence of postoperative supraventricular tachyarrhythmias. The magnitude of this benefit can be estimated to be a near 50% decrease in the incidence of postoperative atrial fibrillation. Therefore, patients receiving beta blockers before coronary bypass surgery should have their preoperative regimen continued until the day of surgery to avoid life threatening ventricular arrhythmias, decrease the incidence of perioperative myocardial infarction and reduce the incidence of postoperative atrial fibrillation. After the operation, the beta blocker therapy should be re-instituted early, within 6 to 12 hours, in hemodynamically stable patients. This approach will decrease the total incidence of postoperative complications by decreasing the episodes of clinically significant atrial fibrillation. Patients scheduled for coronary bypass surgery that are not taking beta blockers before the surgery should have antiadrenergic therapy started preferably 24 to 48 hours before the operation to allow for some antiadrenergic activity to be present in the immediate postoperative period when it helps to blunt the perioperative hyperadrenergic response. Regardless of whether the therapy was started before the surgery, patients will benefit from the early administration of beta blocker therapy for the prevention of postoperative atrial fibrillation.

Even though continuation of preoperative oral beta blockade until the day of surgery and early postoperative reinstitution are beneficial, the same cannot be said about routine use of intravenous antiadrenergic agents immediately before and during the operation. This aggressive use of beta blockers decreases the myocardial oxygen consumption during the intubation and induction of anesthesia period as measured by the rate-pressure product, but this effect does not translate into a clinical benefit as the incidence of perioperative hypotension and bradyarrhythmias increases[13]. Therefore, the use of intravenous beta blockers, either immediately before the surgery or intraoperatively, should be limited to situations in which it is clinically indicated.

The choice of what beta blocking agent to use does not appear nearly as important as the decision to prescribe a beta blocker before and early after the operation. Most of the experience has been accumulated with propranolol but other agents like atenolol and metoprolol, that are more commonly prescribed for the management of angina, are also effective and safe. Continuation of the agent that was used before the surgery, particularly in patients that were already taking a beta blocker at home, is a practical approach since it may ease the transition for continued treatment once the patient is discharged from the intensive care unit and the hospital. The dosage to be used is dictated by the postoperative clinical scenario. In patients that are normotensive or hypertensive the dosage tolerated before the surgery should be reached within 24 to 48 hours after the surgery. Other patients should have the beta blocker therapy started in a lower dose as soon as hemodynamic stability is achieved and then have the dose increased as tolerated with the goal of reaching the preoperative regimen as soon as clinically feasible.

6. Prophylaxis Following Non-coronary Cardiac Surgery

The role of beta blockers for the prevention of postoperative atrial fibrillation in patients undergoing cardiac procedures other than coronary bypass surgery is not well established. Most of the trials discussed above excluded patients undergoing a procedure other than bypass surgery and none of the above trials recruited patients undergoing exclusively a non-coronary bypass procedure. The incidence of postoperative atrial fibrillation after cardiac surgeries other than isolated coronary bypass exceeds 30% in most reports and in some groups, such as those undergoing concomitant mitral valve and bypass surgery, the incidence can be higher than 60% [35-37]. The high occurrence of postoperative atrial fibrillation after non-coronary cardiac surgery may be related to the increased age of some of this patients (i.e. elderly patients with aortic stenosis) as well as the higher incidence of preoperative paroxysmal or chronic atrial fibrillation in others, as in patients with mitral valve disease [38,39]. Although this high incidence of postoperative atrial fibrillation makes them attractive candidates for testing prophylactic strategies, it may reflect that the incidence of atrial fibrillation in this population is more related to the extent of the underlying cardiac condition than to the events directly related to the operation. Conversely, the value of preventing postoperative atrial fibrillation may be less in patients that already have an indication for anticoagulation therapy irrespective of the presence or absence of atrial fibrillation. Indeed, one of the benefits of preventing atrial fibrillation after bypass surgery is the avoidance of such therapy for the prevention of postoperative stroke [40]. It is reasonable to expect based on the above trials that when near normal or normal left ventricular function is present before the operation postoperative beta blockers would be well tolerated and it could be useful in certain group of patients. Whether the routine use of beta blocker therapy in all patients is useful for the prevention of postoperative atrial fibrillation after non-coronary surgery remains to be proved.

References

1. Faulkner SL, Hopkins JT, Boerth RC, et al. Time required for complete recovery from chronic propranolol therapy. N Engl J M 1973;289:607-9.
2. Jones EL, Kaplan JA, Dorney ER, et al. Propranolol therapy in patients undergoing myocardial revascularization. Am J Cardiol 1976;38:696-700.
3. Viljoen JF, Estafanous FG, Kellner GA. Propranolol and cardiac surgery. J Thorac Cardiovasc Surg 1972;64:826-30.
4. Diaz RG, Somberg JC, Freeman E, et al. Withdrawal of propranolol and myocardial infarction. Lancet 1973;1:1068.
5. Miller RR, Olson HG, Amsterdam EA, et al. Propranolol-withdrawal rebound phenomenon. Exacerbation of coronary events after abrupt cessation of anti anginal therapy. N Engl J Med 1975;293:416-8.
6. Salazar C, Frishman W, Freidman S et al. Beta-blockade therapy for supraventricular tachyarrhythmias after coronary surgery: a propranolol withdrawal syndrome? Angiology 1979;30:816-9.
7. Boudolas H. Snyder GL, Lewis RP, et al. Safety and rationale for continuation of propranolol therapy during coronary bypass operation. Ann Thorac Surg 1978;26:222-29.
8. Kirsh MM, Douglas MB, Jackson AP, et al. Myocardial revascularization in patients receiving long-term propranolol therapy. Ann Thorac Surg 1978;25:117-21.
9. Oka Y, Frisman W, Becker RM. Clinical pharmacology of the new beta-adrenergic blocking drugs. Part 10. Beta-adrenoreceptor blockade and coronary artery surgery. Am Heart J 1980;99:255-69.
10. Stephenson LW, MacVaugh H, Tomasselo DN, Josephson ME. Propranolol for prevention of postoperative cardiac arrhythmias: a randomized study. Ann Thorac Surg 1980;29:113-6.
11. Mohr R, Smolonsky A, Goor DA. Prevention of supraventricular tachyarrhythmias with low-dose propranolol after coronary bypass. J Thorac Cardiovasc Surg 1981;81:841-5.
12. Silverman NA, Wright R, Levitsky S. Efficacy of low dose propranolol in preventing postoperative supraventricular tachyarrhythmias: a prospective, randomized study. Ann Surg 1982;196:194-7.
13. Abel RM, Van Gelder H. Pores IH, Liguori J, Gielchinski I, Parsonnet V. Continued propranolol administration following coronary bypass surgery: antiarrhythmic effects. Arch Surg 1983;118:727-31.

14. Ivey MF, Ivey TD, Bailey WW, Williams DB, Hessel EA II, Miller DW Jr. Influence of propranolol on supraventricular tachycardia early after coronary ravascularization: a randomized trial. J Thorac Cardiovasc Surg 1983;85:214-8.

15. Hammond JW Jr, Wood AJ, Prager RL, Wood M, Muirhead J, Bender HW Jr. Perioperative beta blockade with propranolol: Reduction in myocardial oxygen demands and incidence of atrial and ventricular arrhythmias. Ann Thorac Surg 1984;38:363-7.

16. Matangi MF, Neutze JM, Graham KJ, Hill DG, Kerr AR, Barrat-Boyes BG. Arrhythmia prophylaxis after aorta-coronary bypass. The effect of mini dose propranolol. J Thorac Cardiovasc Surg 1985;89:439-43

17. Martinussen HJ, Lolk A, Szczepanski C, Alstrup P. Supraventricular tachyarrhythmias after coronary bypass surgery - a double-blind randomized trial of prophylactic low dose propranolol. Thorac Cardiovasc Surg 1988;36:206-7.

18. Shafei H, Nashef SA, Turner MA, Brian WH. Does low-dose propranol reduce the incidence of supraventricular tachyarrhythmias following myocardial revascularization? A clinical study. Thorac Cardiovasc Surg 1988;36:202-5.

19. Ormerod OJM, McGregor CGA, Stone DL, Wisbey C, Petch MC. Arrhythmias after coronary bypass surgery. Br. Heart J 1984;51:618-21.

20. Rubin DA, Nieminski KE, Reed GE, Herman MV. Predictors, prevention, and long term prognosis of atrial fibrillation after coronary artery bypass graft operations. J Thorac Cardiovasc Surg 1987;94:331-5.

22. Mills SA, Poole GV, Breyer RH et al. Digoxin and propranolol in the prophylaxis of dysrythmias after coronary bypass grafting. Circulation 1983;68: Suppl II:II-222-II-225.

23. Kendall MJ. Are selective beta-adrenoreceptor blocking drugs an advantage? J R Coll Phys Lond 1981;15:33-40.

24. White HD, Antman EM, Glynn MA, et al. Efficacy and safety of timolol for prevention of supraventricular tachyarrhythmias after coronary bypass surgery. Circulation 1984;70:479-84.

25. Vecht RJ, Nicolaides EP, Ikweuke JK, Liassides C, Cleary J, Cooper WB. Incidence and prevention of supraventricular tachycardias after coronary bypass surgery. Int J Cardiol 1986;13:125-34.

26. Daudon P, Corcos T, Gandjbakhch I, Levasseur JP, Cabrol A, Cabrol C. Prevention of atrial fibrillation or flutter by acebutolol after coronary bypass grafting. Am J Cardiol 1986;58:933-6.

27. Materne P, Larbuisson R, Collignon P, Limet R, Kulbertus H. Prevention by acebutolol of rhythm disorders following coronary artery bypass surgery. Int J Cardiol 1985;8:275-283.

28. Khuri SF, Okike N, Josa M et al. Efficacy of nadolol in preventing supraventricular tachycardia after coronary bypass grafting. Am J Cardiol 1987;60:51D-58D.

29. Lamb RK, Prabhakar G, Thorpe JAC, Smith S, Norton R, Dyde JA. The use of atenolol in the prevention of supraventricular arrhythmias following coronary artery surgery. Eur Heart J 1988;9:32-6.

30. Matangi MM, Strickland J, Garbe GJ, et al. Atenolol for the prevention of arrhythmias following coronary artery bypass grafting. Can J Cardiol 1989;5:229-34.

31. Janssen J, Loomans L, Harink L, et al. Prevention and treatment of supraventricular tachycardia shortly after coronary bypass grafting: a randomized open trial. Angiology 1986;37:601-9.

32. Kowey PR, Taylor JE, Rials SJ, Marinchak RA. Meta-analysis of the effectiveness of prophylactic drug therapy in preventing supraventricular arrhythmia early after coronary artery bypass grafting. Am J Cardiol 1992;69:963-65.

33. Andrews TC, Reimold SC, Berlin JA, Antman EA. Prevention of supraventricular arrhythmias after coronary artery bypass surgery. A meta-analysis of randomized control trials. Circulation 1991;84:Suppl III:III-236-III-244.

34. Yusuf S, Peto R, Lewis J, Collins R, Sleight P. Beta blockade during and after myocardial infarction: an overview of the randomized trials. Prog Cardiovasc Dis 1985;27:335-71.

35. Bush HL Jr., Gelband H, Hoffman BF, Malm JR. Electrophysiological basis for supraventricular arrhythmias following surgical procedures for aortic stenosis. Arch Surg 1971;103:620-5.

36. Hoie J, Forfang K. Arrhythmias and conduction disturbances following aortic valve implantation. Scand J Thor Cardiovasc Surg 1980;14:177-83.

37. Creswell LL, Rosembloom M, Schuessler RB, Cox JL. Atrial arrhythmias after cardiac surgical procedure: An updated examination of risk factors. J Am Coll Cardiol 1993;21:122A.abstract.

38. Douglas P, Hishfeld JW Jr, Edmunds LH. Clinical correlates of postoperative atrial fibrillation. Circulation 1984;70:Suppl II:II-165.abstract.

39. Mathew JP, Parks R, Savino JS, et al. Atrial fibrillation following coronary artery bypass graft surgery. Predictors, outcome, and resource utilization. JAMA 1996;276:300-6.

40. Lauer MS, Eagle KA, Buckley MJ, DeSanctis RW. Atrial fibrillation following coronary bypass surgery. Prog Cardiovasc Dis 1989;5:367-78.

7 ANTIARRHYTHMIC THERAPY TO PREVENT ATRIAL FIBRILLATION AFTER CARDIAC SURGERY

Bradley P. Knight, MD and Fred Morady, MD,
The University of Michigan Medical Center,
Ann Arbor, MI

1. Introduction

Cardiac surgery and the postoperative state are associated with increased catecholamine levels [1]. Therefore, beta-blockers are logical agents to prevent atrial fibrillation in this setting. Indeed, many trials have shown a benefit with prophylactic beta-blockade [2-9]. However, the data regarding beta-blockers must be interpreted with caution. Some of the apparent benefit of beta-blockers may be explained by beta-blocker withdrawal in patients assigned to placebo. In addition, many of the beta-blocker trials excluded patients with left ventricular dysfunction and obstructive lung disease, and patients undergoing concomitant valvular surgery. Because of the limitations of beta-blockers and because there is a significant incidence of postoperative atrial fibrillation despite beta-blocker prophylaxis, other pharmacological approaches to prevent postoperative atrial fibrillation have been investigated.

This chapter reviews the data regarding the use of antiarrhythmic drugs other than beta-blockers to prevent atrial fibrillation after cardiac surgery. The ideal prophylactic agent would reduce the number of patients who develop postoperative atrial fibrillation, reduce the number of episodes per patient, provide ventricular rate control among patients who develop atrial fibrillation, be applicable to all patients, and have a low side effect profile. Despite the availability of several antiarrhythmic drugs for the treatment of atrial fibrillation, only a few have been evaluated as prophylactic agents in the postoperative setting; these include digitalis [10-13], magnesium [14-15], verapamil [16], procainamide [17], sotalol [18-22], and amiodarone [23-26] (Table).

Drug	Regimen	Control	Yr	N	AF Incidence Control	Drug	%▲	P
Digoxin[10]	Preop load→0.25 mg/d	Placebo	76	120	26%	6%	-77%	<0.01
Digoxin[11]	Preop load→0.25 mg/d	Placebo	79	140	11%	28%	+255%	<0.05
Digoxin[12]	Postop load→0.25 mg/d	Placebo	81	407	15%	2%	-87%	<0.01
Digoxin[13]	Postop load→0.25 mg/d	Placebo	82	182	72%	5%	-93%	<0.01
Magnesium[14]	712 meq IV/4d	Placebo	91	99	28%	14%	-50%	NS
Magnesium[15]	140 meq IV/2d	Placebo	93	140	26%	29%	+12%	NS
Verapamil[16]	320 mg/d PO	Placebo	85	200	23%	14%	-39%	<0.1
Procainamide[17]	2mg/min IV	Placebo	93	46	38%	18%	-53%	0.2
Sotalol[18]	240 mg/d	Placebo	86	91	36%	2%	-94%	<0.01
Sotalol[18]	240 mg/d	Metoprolol 150 mg/d	86	80	15%	2%	-87%	<0.05
Sotalol[19]	120 mg/d	Propranolol 40 mg/d	90	140	18%	14%	-22%	NS
Sotalol[19]	240 mg/d	Propranolol 80 mg/d	90	289	14%	11%	-21%	NS
Sotalol[20]	160 mg/d	Placebo	91	300	33%	16%	-52%	<0.01
Sotalol[21]	320 mg/d	Routine*	92	101	29%	10%	-66%	0.03
Sotalol[22]	120 mg/d	Metoprolol 75 mg/d	98	191	32%	16%	-50%	<0.01
Amiodarone[23]	4.5gm IV/4d	Placebo	91	77	21%	5%	-76%	<0.05
Amiodarone[24]	1.5gm IV/1d→600 mg/d	Placebo	93	120	20%	8%	-60%	0.07
Amiodarone[25]	2gm IV/2d	Placebo	98	300	47%	35%	-26%	0.03
Amiodarone[26]	4.2 gm PO/7d→200 mg/d	Placebo	97	124	53%	25%	-53%	<0.01

*Routine practice included beta-blockers in 40% of patients. Abbreviations: AF = atrial fibrillation; d = days; IV = intravenously; N = number of patients; NS = not statistically significant; PO = orally; preop = preoperatively; postop = postoperatively; yr = year; ▲ = change.

2. Digoxin

Digitalis was advocated in the past for the prevention of supraventricular arrhythmias after coronary bypass surgery. Three studies in the late 1970's and early 1980's demonstrated a significant reduction in the incidence of atrial fibrillation with digoxin when given as an intravenous load preoperatively or postoperatively [10,12,13]. However, a fourth study by Tyras et al [11] found that digoxin more than doubled the incidence of atrial fibrillation. The findings of Tyras et al, the concern that postoperative myocardial sensitivity might lead to digoxin toxicity, and evidence that digoxin does not convert atrial fibrillation [27], have discouraged the prophylactic use of digoxin.

3. Calcium Channel Blockers

There is increasing evidence that intracellular calcium overload occurs during atrial fibrillation and is associated with a shortening of atrial refractoriness [28,29]. This so-called electrical remodeling promotes recurrent episodes of atrial fibrillation, but can be attenuated by verapamil [30]. Therefore, calcium-channel antagonists may be useful in the prevention of atrial fibrillation. Calcium-blockers might be expected to not only reduce the number of patients who develop atrial fibrillation, but also to reduce the number of episodes per patient and control the ventricular response during atrial fibrillation. Verapamil was evaluated as a prophylactic agent using a daily oral dose of 320 mg given postoperatively [16]. Verapamil resulted in a 39% reduction in number of patients who developed atrial fibrillation but was associated with a 20% discontinuation rate. Thirteen percent of the patients treated with verapamil developed hypotension and/or pulmonary edema compared to 1% of patients treated with placebo (p<0.001). Therefore, although calcium channel blockers may have theoretical advantages, they appear to be associated with unacceptable adverse hemodynamic effects. Future studies with calcium-channel blockers are unlikely given the increasing concern that the use of calcium channel blockers, with the exception of some of the newer, more vascular-specific agents [31,32], may be detrimental in patients with ischemic cardiomyopathy [33,34].

4. Magnesium Supplementation

Magnesium is a required cofactor for the maintenance of normal cardiac transmembrane sodium and potassium gradients. Hypomagnesemia occurs after cardiac surgery and was found in a study by Kalman et al to be an independent predictor of postoperative atrial fibrillation [35]. Factors thought to contribute to the postoperative reduction in serum magnesium concentrations include hemodilution, diuretic use, and catecholamine stimulation.

Two groups of investigators attempted to use magnesium supplementation to prevent atrial fibrillation [14,15]. In parallel with trials using prophylactic magnesium for ventricular arrhythmias in the setting of myocardial infarction [36-38], initially encouraging results were not supported by larger subsequent trials. The first placebo-controlled study using magnesium supplementation included 99 patients and administered a total of 712 meq of intravenous magnesium sulfate over the first 4 postoperative days [14]. Magnesium resulted in a 50% reduction in the incidence of atrial fibrillation from 28% to 14%, although the difference did not reach statistical significance. In a second study of 140 patients, 140 meq of intravenous magnesium sulfate was administered over the first 2 postoperative days and no difference was found in the incidence of atrial fibrillation in the treated group compared to the placebo (29% vs 26%; p=NS), despite confirmation of serum magnesium repletion [15]. In addition, the incidence of atrial fibrillation was found to have a direct correlation with serum magnesium levels, suggesting a proarrhythmic effect. Therefore, although hypomagnesemia is present following bypass surgery, it may only reflect increased sympathetic tone and its correction does not prevent atrial fibrillation.

5. Procainamide

Procainamide is the only class I antiarrhythmic drug that has been evaluated as a prophylactic agent. A pilot study comparing procainamide to placebo in 46 patients was published by Laub et al in 1993 [17]. Procainamide was associated with a 53% reduction in the incidence of atrial fibrillation, but the difference did not reach statistical significance (p=0.2). However, the total number of episodes of atrial fibrillation was significantly reduced in the group that received procainamide. Larger trials have not been published.

6. Sotalol

Sotalol is a class III antiarrhythmic drug. The combined potassium-channel blocking and nonselective beta-blocking properties of sotalol make it an ideal agent for postoperative atrial fibrillation. In addition, the reverse use-dependent effect of sotalol, which results in more potent effects at slower atrial rates, suggest that sotalol may be more effective in the prevention of atrial fibrillation than in its conversion. Five studies using various sotalol dosages and types of control groups have been published [18-22]. The first trial, published in 1986, compared sotalol 240 mg/day to both metoprolol 150 mg/day and to placebo [18]. Metoprolol significantly reduced the incidence of atrial fibrillation to 15% compared to 36% in the placebo group (p<0.01), but sotalol further reduced the incidence to 2% (p<0.05 compared to metoprolol). A more recent trial also found sotalol 120 mg/day to be more effective than metoprolol 75 mg/day [22].

One trial compared sotalol to propranolol and was designed with 4 treatment groups: sotalol 120 mg/day, sotalol 240 mg/day, propranolol 80 mg/day, and propranolol 40 mg/day [19]. Efficacy was similar among groups, but the group that received high-dose sotalol had a much higher incidence of side effects than those who received low-dose sotalol. Sotalol has been compared to placebo at a dose of 160 mg/day [21], and to the standard local practice, which included beta-blockers in 40% of the patients, at a dose of 320 mg/day [22]. Both studies found a significant benefit of sotalol compared to control, but the discontinuation rate was 10% when 320 mg/day was used compared to 1% when 160 mg/day was used.

In summary, data regarding the use of sotalol for the prevention of postoperative atrial fibrillation suggest that sotalol is more effective than the cardioselective beta-blocker metoprolol, but is comparable to the nonselective beta-blocker propranolol. Low doses of sotalol in the range of 120-160 mg/day appear to be as effective as 240-360 mg/day, but are better tolerated. Although the incidence of torsades de pointes was low in these studies, sotalol has significant negative inotropic effects and should be used with caution in patients with symptomatic heart failure following open heart surgery.

7. Amiodarone

Amiodarone is a class III antiarrhythmic drug with many properties that make it an excellent candidate for postoperative atrial fibrillation prophylaxis. Amiodarone is effective in maintaining sinus rhythm in patients with history of atrial fibrillation [39-41], has anti-ischemic properties [42,43], has minimal negative inotropic effects [44], and has a low risk of proarrhythmia in patients with structural heart disease [45].

Three studies have compared the postoperative administration of amiodarone to placebo. Hohnloser, et al administered a total of 4.5 gm of intravenous amiodarone over 4 days and found a reduction in the incidence of atrial fibrillation from 21% to 5% (p<0.05) [23]. Butler, et al infused 1.5 gm of amiodarone intravenously during the first postoperative day and then administered 600 mg/day orally during the next 5 days (for a total of 4.5 gm) [24]. Although a 60% reduction in the incidence of atrial fibrillation was observed, the difference was not statistically significant (p=0.07). Bradycardia was noted in 78% of the patients, but was of sufficient severity to warrant discontinuation in only 1 patient.

Preliminary results from the Amiodarone Reduces CABG Hospitalization (ARCH) trial were presented at the 47th Annual Scientific Session of the American College of Cardiology [24]. Three hundred patients were randomized to receive either 2 gm of intravenous amiodarone or placebo during the first 2 postoperative days. Amiodarone resulted in a significant decrease in atrial fibrillation from 47% to 35% (p=0.03). The duration of hospitalization tended to be shorter for patients treated with amiodarone compared to placebo, but the difference was not statistically significant (7.5 vs. 8.2 days; p=0.3). Amiodarone did not significantly reduce the ventricular rate among patients who developed atrial fibrillation. There was no significant morbidity or mortality attributable to amiodarone.

A recent randomized, double-blinded, placebo-controlled study evaluated the prophylactic use of preoperative oral amiodarone among patients who were scheduled for elective cardiac surgery [26]. Exclusion criteria included the use of class I or III antiarrhythmic drugs, untreated thyroid disease, liver enzyme elevation, resting heart rate less than 50 bpm, and uncontrolled heart failure. The study population included 124 patients and differed from other trials in that a high proportion of patients underwent cardiac valve surgery, either alone (40%) or with bypass grafting (18%). The 64 patients randomized to receive amiodarone were given 600 mg/day for 7 days prior to surgery, followed by 200 mg/day postoperatively until discharge from the hospital. The mean total outpatient dose was 4.8 gm. A postoperative episode of atrial fibrillation was counted if it lasted more than 5 minutes based on telemetry data. A single-lead rhythm strip was recorded by a visiting nurse one week following hospital discharge, and a 12-lead ECG was performed in an outpatient clinic 3 to 5 weeks following discharge.

Outpatient compliance by pill count was excellent and the study drug was discontinued in only 1 patient in the amiodarone group and 1 patient in the placebo group. Amiodarone resulted in an overall decrease in the incidence of atrial fibrillation (25% vs. 53%; p<0.01) with both a decrease in the incidence of in-hospital atrial fibrillation (23% vs. 42%; p=0.03), as well as atrial fibrillation occurring after discharge (2% vs. 12%; p=0.03). Furthermore, patients who were treated with amiodarone had a significantly shorter hospital length of stay compared to placebo (6.5±2.6 vs. 7.9±4.3 days; p=0.04), and a substantial cost savings of approximately $8,000 per patient. Amiodarone resulted in no significant difference in intraoperative complications, hospital major morbidity, malignant ventricular arrhythmias, or mortality.

In summary, postoperative intravenous amiodarone appears to be safe and effective in reducing the incidence of postoperative atrial fibrillation, but is associated with a high incidence of bradycardia. Amiodarone appears to be more effective when doses of approximately 4 gm are given compared to 2 gm. A preoperative strategy using oral amiodarone appears to be effective and well tolerated. The main limitation of a preoperative amiodarone regimen is the requirement for sufficient time prior to surgery to allow for adequate drug administration, which excludes patients who undergo cardiac surgery on an emergent or semi-emergent basis.

8. Future Prospects

Targeted drug delivery to the atria may be safer and more effective than systemic drug delivery for the prevention of postoperative atrial fibrillation. Direct pericardial installation of antiarrhythmic drugs at the time of surgery is a potential method for targeting drug delivery. Amiodarone delivered into the pericardial sac of dogs results in high atrial tissue amiodarone concentrations despite low serum concentrations, increases atrial refractoriness, and suppresses the ability to induce atrial fibrillation with pacing [46]. Another potential method for targeting drug delivery is the use of drug-coated epicardial wires. The use of controlled delivery devices has been applied to the area of antiarrhythmic drug therapy [47], but is currently not available for the prevention of postoperative atrial fibrillation.

Combinations of pharmacologic and nonpharmacologic therapies may be required to cause a major impact on the problem of postoperative atrial fibrillation. The use of a class III antiarrhythmic drugs with biatrial pacing is an attractive option.

8. Conclusion

Beta-blockers may reduce the incidence of atrial fibrillation, but several studies have had conflicting results. Digoxin loading and magnesium supplementation appear to be ineffective. Procainamide may be effective but has been inadequately studied. Verapamil is associated with a high incidence of adverse hemodynamic effects. One week of oral preoperative amiodarone is highly effective and well tolerated. For patients who undergo nonelective cardiac surgery, low dose oral sotalol or intravenous amiodarone are reasonable regimens to prevent atrial fibrillation. Potential prophylactic treatments in the future include targeted drug therapy or the combined use of pharmacologic and nonpharmacologic agents.

References

1. Kalman JM, Munawar M, Howes LG, Louis WJ, Buxton BF, Gutteridge G, Tonkin AM. Atrial fibrillation after coronary artery bypass grafting is associated with sympathetic activation. Ann Thorac Surg 1995;60:1709-15.
2. Daudon P, Corcos T, Gandjbakhch I, Levasseur J, Cabrol A, Cabrol C. Prevention of atrial fibrillation or flutter by acebutolol after coronary bypass grafting. Am J Cardiol 1986;58:933-36.
3. Silverman NA, Wright R, Levitsky S. Efficacy of low-dose propranolol in preventing postoperative supraventricular tachyarrhythmias. A prospective, randomized study. Ann Surg 1982;196:194-97.
4. Abel RM, van Gelder HM, Pores IH, Liguori J, Gielchinsky I, Parsonnet V. Continued propranolol administration following coronary bypass surgery. Arch Surg 1983;118:727-31.
5. Martinussen HJ, Lolk A, Szczepanski C, Alstrup P. Supraventricular tachyarrhythmias after coronary bypass surgery – A double blind randomized trial of prophylactic low dose propranolol. Thorac cardiovasc Surgeon 1988;36:206-7.
6. Ivey MF, Ivey TD, Bailey WW, Williams DB, Hessel EA, Miller DW. Influence of propranolol on supraventricular tachycardia early after coronary artery revascularization. J Thorac Cardiovasc Surg 1983; 85:214-18.
7. Shafie H, Nashef SAM, Turner MA, Bain WH. Does low-dose propranolol reduce the incidence of supraventricular tachyarrhythmias following myocardial revascularization? – A clinical study. Thorac cardiovasc Surgeon 1988;36:202-5.
8. White HD, Antman EM, Glynn MA, Collins JJ, Cohn LH, Shemin RJ, Friedman PL. Efficacy and safety of timolol for prevention of supraventricular tachyarrhythmias after coronary artery bypass surgery. Circulation 1984;70:479-84.
9. Lamb RK, Prabhakar G, Thorpe JAC, Smith S, Norton R, Dyde JA. The use of atenolol in the prevention of supraventricular arrhythmias following coronary artery surgery. Eur Heart J 1988;9:32-36.
10. Johnson LW, Dickstein RA, Fruehan CT, Kane P, Potts JL, Smulyan H, Webb WR, Eich RH. Prophylactic digitalization for coronary artery bypass surgery. Circulation 1976;53:819-22.

11. Tyras DH, Stothert JC, Kaiser GC, Barner HB, Codd JE, Willman VL. Supraventricular tachyarrhythmias after myocardial revascularization: A randomized trial of prophylactic digitalization. J Thorac Cardiovasc Surg. 1979;77:310-4.

12. Csicsko JF, Schatzlein MH, King RD. Immediate postoperative digitalization in the prophylaxis of supraventricular arrhythmias following coronary artery bypass. J Thorac Cardiovasc Surg 1981;81:419-22.

13. Chee TP, Prakash NS, Desser KB, Benchimol A. Postoperative supraventricular arrhythmias and the role of prophylactic digoxin in cardiac surgery. Am Heart J 1982;104:974-7.

14. Fanning WJ, Thomas CS, Roach A, Tomichek R, Alford WC, Stoney WS. Prophylaxis of atrial fibrillation with magnesium sulfate after coronary artery bypass grafting. Ann Thorac Surg 1991;52:529-33.

15. Parikka H, Toivonen L, Pellinen T, Verkkala K, Jarvinen A, Nieminen MS. The influence of intravenous magnesium sulphate on the occurrence of atrial fibrillation after coronary artery by-pass operation. Eur Heart J 1993;14:251-.

16. Davison R, Hartz R, Kaplan K, Parker M, Feiereisel P, Michaelis L. Prophylaxis of supraventricular tachyarrhythmia after coronary bypass surgery with oral verapamil: A randomized, double-blind trial. Ann Thorac Surg 1985;39:336-9.

17. Laub GW, Janeira L, Muralidharan S, Riebman JB, Chen C, Neary M, Fernandez J, Adkins MS, McGrath LB. Prophylactic procainamide for prevention of atrial fibrillation after coronary artery bypass grafting: A prospective, double-blind, randomized, placebo-controlled pilot study. Critic Care Med 1993;21:1474-8.

18. Janssen J, Loomans L, Harink J, Taams M, Brunninkhuis L, van der Starre P, Kootstra G. Prevention and treatment of supraventricular tachycardia shortly after coronary artery bypass grafting: A randomized open trial. J Vasc Dis 1986;37:601-9.

19. Suttorp MJ, Kingma JH, Tjon Joe Gin RM, van Hemel NM, Koomen EM, Defauw JA, Adan AJM, Ernst SM. Efficacy and safety of low- and high-dose sotalol versus propranolol in the prevention of supraventricular tachyarrhythmias early after coronary artery bypass operations. J Thorac Cardiovas Surg 1990;100:921-6.

20. Suttorp MJ, Kingma JH, Peels HOJ, Koomen EM, Tifssen JGP, van Hemel NM, Defauw JAM, Ernst SMPG. Effectiveness of sotalol in preventing supraventricular tachyarrhythmias shortly after coronary artery bypass grafting. Am J Cardiol 1991;68:1163-69.

21. Nystrom U, Edvardsson N, Berggren H. Pizzarelli GP, Radegran K. Oral sotalol reduces the incidence of atrial fibrillation after coronary artery bypass surgery. Thorac cardiovasc Surgeon 1993; 41:34-37.

22. Parikka H, Toivonen L, Heikkila, L, Virtanen K, Jarvinan A. Comparison of sotalol and metoprolol in the prevention of atrial fibrillation after coronary artery bypass surgery. J Cardiovasc Pharmacol 1998;31:67-73.

23. Hohnloser SH, Meinertz T, Dammbacher T, Steiert K, Jamhnchen E, Zehender M, Fraedrich G, Just H. Electrocardiographic and antiarrhythmic effects of intravenous amiodarone: Results of a prospective, placebo-controlled study. Am Heart J 1991;121:89-95.

24. Butler J, Harriss DR, Sinclair M, Westaby S. Amiodarone prophylaxis for tachycardias after coronary artery surgery: A randomised, double blind, placebo controlled trial. Br Heart J 1993;70:56-60.

25. Guarnieri T. Amiodarone Reduces CABG Hospitalization (ARCH) trial. Presented as a Late Breaking Clinical Trial at the 47th Annual Scientific Session of the American College of Cardiology. March 1998.

26. Daoud EG, Strickberger SA, Man KC, Goyal R, Deeb GM, Bolling SF, Pagani FD, Bitar C, Meissner MD, Morady F. Preoperative amiodarone as prophylaxis against atrial fibrillation after heart surgery. NEJM 1997;337:1785-91.

27. The Digitalis in Acute Atrial Fibrillation (DAAF) Trial Group. Intravenous digoxin in acute atrial fibrillation. Results of a randomized, placebo-controlled multicentre trial in 239 patients. European Heart Journal 1997;18:649-54.

28. Wijffels MCEF, Kirchhof CJHJ, Dorland R, Allessie MA. Atrial fibrillation begets atrial fibrillation: a study in awake chronically instrumented goats. Circulation 1995;92:1954-1968.

29. Daoud EG, Bogun F, Goyal R, Harvey M, Man KC, Strickberger SA, Morady F. Effect of atrial fibrillation on atrial refractoriness in humans. Circulation 1996;94:1600-1606.

30. Daoud EG. Knight BP. Weiss R. Bahu M. Paladino W. Goyal R. Man KC. Strickberger SA. Morady F. Effect of verapamil and procainamide on atrial fibrillation-induced electrical remodeling in humans. Circulation 1997;5:1542-5019.

31. Packer M, O'Connor CM, Ghali JK, et al, for the Prospective Randomized Amlodipine Survival Evaluation Study Group. Effect of amlodipine on morbidity and mortality in severe chronic heart failure. NEJM. 1996;335:1107-1114.

32. Cohn JN, Ziesche S, Smith R, Anand I, Dunkman WB, Loeb H, Cintron G, Boden W, Baruch L, Rochin P, Loss L. Effect of the calcium antagonist felodipine as supplementary vasodilator therapy in patients with chronic heart failure treated with enalapril. V-HeFT III. Vasodilator-Heart Failure Trial (V-HeFT) Study Group. Circulation 1997;96:856-63.

33. The Multicenter Diltiazem Postinfarction Trial Research Group. The effect of diltiazem on mortality and reinfarction after myocardial infarction. NEJM. 1988;319:385-392.

34. Cheng JW. Behar L. Calcium channel blockers: association with myocardial infarction, mortality, and cancer. [Review]. Clinical Therapeutics 1997;19:1255-68.

35. Aranki SF, Shaw DP, Adams DH, Rizzo RJ, Couper GS, VanderVliet M, Collins JJ, Cohn LH, Burstin HR. Predictors of atrial fibrillation after coronary artery surgery. Current trends and impact on hospital resources. Circulation 1996;94:390-97.

36. Woods KL, Fletcher S, Roffe C, Haider Y. Intravenous magnesium sulphate in suspected acute myocardial infarction: results of the second Leicester Intravenous Magnesium Intervention Trial (LIMIT-2). Lancet 1992;339:1553-58.

37. ISIS-4 (Fourth International Study of Infarct Survival) Collaborative Group. ISIS-4: a randomised factorial trial assessing early oral captopril, oral mononitrate, and intravenous magnesium sulphate in 58,050 patients with suspected acute myocardial infarction. Lancet 1995;345:669-85.

38. Baxter GF, Sumeray MS, Walker JM. Infarct size and magnesium: insights into LIMIT-2 and ISIS-4 from experimental studies. Lancet 1996; 348: 1424-26.

39. Chun S, Sager P, Stevenson W, Nademanee K, Middlekauff H, Singh B. Amiodarone is highly effective in maintaining NSR in refractory atrial fibrillation/flutter. J Am Coll Cardiol 1993;21:203A.

40. Middlekauff HR, Wiener I, Stevenson WG. Low-dose amiodarone for atrial fibrillation. Am J Cardiol 1993;72:75F-81F.

41. Gosselink ATM, Crijns HJGM, Van Gelder IC, Hillige H, Wiesfeld ACP, Lie KI. Low-dose amiodarone for maintenance of sinus rhythm after cardioversion of atrial fibrillation or flutter. JAMA 1992;267:3289-93.

42. Mason JW. Amiodarone. N Engl J Med 1987;316:455-66.

43. Hondeghem LM. Class III agents: amiodarone, bretylium, and sotalol. In: Zipes DP, Jalife J, eds. Cardiac electrophysiology: from cell to bedside. 2nd ed. Philadelphia: W.B. Saunders, 1995:1330-6.

44. Hamer AWF, Arkles LB, Johns JA. Beneficial effects of low dose amiodarone in patients with congestive cardiac failure: a placebo-controlled trial. J Am Coll Cardiol 1989;14:1768-74.

45. Nicklas JM, McKenna WJ, Stewart RA, et al. Prospective, double-blind, placebo-controlled trial of low-dose amiodarone in patients with severe heart failure and asymptomatic frequent ventricular ectopy. Am Heart J 1991;122:1016-21.

46. Ayers GM, Rho TH, Ben-David J, Besch HR Jr, Zipes DP. Amiodarone instilled into the canine pericardial sac migrates transmurally to produce electrophysiologic effects and suppress atrial fibrillation. Journal of Cardiovascular Electrophysiology 1996;7:713-21.

47. Labhasetwar V. Levy RJ. Novel delivery of antiarrhythmic agents. (Review) Clinical Pharmacokinetics 1995;29:1-5.

8 NONPHARMACOLOGIC TREATMENT OF POSTOPERATIVE ATRIAL FIBRILLATION

Richard J. Lewis, MD, PhD and
Jonathan S. Steinberg, MD,
St. Luke's-Roosevelt Hospital Center and
Columbia University College of Physicians and
Surgeons, New York, NY

1. Background

Atrial fibrillation (AF) remains one of the more serious and common postoperative complications in patients undergoing coronary artery bypass graft (CABG) surgery. An incidence of 10-50% has been reported in numerous studies over the last two decades [1-8, see also chapter 3]. Efforts to prevent postoperative AF have included refinements in intraoperative surgical technique, use of pre-, intra- and postoperative beta-blockers, prophylactic antiarrhythmic drugs, and multiple temporary cardiac pacing strategies.

A number of operative advances including the adoption of continuous cardioplegia [9], retrograde cardioplegia, warm cardioplegia and evolution of the cardioplegia cocktail, while improving myocardial protection, did not significantly alter the incidence of postoperative AF [8, 10-12]. The results of use of amiodarone with oral preoperative loading [13] and low dose IV postoperative infusion [14] are certainly encouraging. However, despite clear benefit of amiodarone, the postoperative incidence of AF was reduced from about 50% to only 25%[13,14].

With the incidence of postoperative AF remaining so high despite the current best pharmacological prophylaxis, additional nonpharmacologic strategies to prevent AF continue to hold great interest.

2. Postoperative Pacing to Prevent Atrial Fibrillation

2.1. Lessons from permanent pacing

Experience gained from permanent pacing may provide insights for prevention of post-CABG AF by temporary pacing. Controversy over whether atrial or ventricular-based pacing mode was most appropriate for the patient with sinus node disease has been present since the introduction of pacing for sick sinus syndrome. While the theoretical benefits of maintaining AV synchrony was certainly appreciated, concern over atrial lead stability [15], rising capture thresholds in the coronary sinus (the only site initially used for atrial pacing) [16] and potential proarrhythmia from atrial leads resulted in early pacing using both AAI and VVI modes [for review, see reference17]. In 1986, Sutton and Kenny reported the difference in AF development in patients with AAI verses VVI pacing modes [18]. Of 410 patients with atrial pacemakers, 3.9% developed AF over 33 months. Of 651 patients with ventricular pacemakers, 22.3% developed AF over 39 months. A few years later, a prospective, nonrandomized trial comparing AAI verses VVI pacing for sick sinus syndrome was published [19]. After a 4-year follow-up period, 47% of the ventricular paced patients developed AF compared to only 7% of those patients paced in the AAI mode. A review of several retrospective studies demonstrated a yearly rate of AF development of 7.5% in patients paced VVI versus only 2.2% for patients paced AAI or DDD [20]. No difference was observed between AAI and DDD modes [17,20]. The possibility that VVI pacing might actually be responsible for causing AF was highlighted by the observation that patients who received VVI pacemakers had a higher incidence of developing AF than patients receiving DVI or DDD pacemakers even if the underlying arrhythmia was heart block and not sinus node disease [21]. The first prospective randomized controlled trial comparing atrial and ventricular pacing in sick sinus syndrome was reported in 1993 [22]. This Danish trial demonstrated a lower likelihood of AF in the AAI/DDD group than in patients paced VVI. Multiple studies have documented similar findings [23-25] although additional larger trials are ongoing [26,27].

2.2. Temporary pacing

The very first attempts at pacing the heart by Zoll in 1952 were external or transthoracic [28]. Although this technique is still utilized for patients with cardiac arrest and bradycardia, the discomfort and unreliability make this mode of pacing inadequate for the routine treatment of post-CABG patients. Transesophageal atrial pacing, first demonstrated by Shafiroff and Linder in 1957 [29], may still be a useful technique for diagnosing arrhythmias and for overdrive pacing to terminate reentrant tachycardias, but is inadequate for routine temporary pacing due to discomfort and lead migration. Furthermore, while fairly reliable for atrial pacing, it is not as successful for ventricular capture [30]. Transvenous pacing has certainly become the preferred means of pacing both for temporary and permanent objectives due to this technique's relative ease and patient comfort as well as reliability and safety. However, in the patient already undergoing open-heart surgery, an even easier and safer means of temporary pacing is available. Thin Teflon-coated wires with the tips bared can easily be sutured to the epicardial surface of the heart and brought through the chest wall for connection to a temporary pacemaker. When temporary pacing is no longer needed, these leads can be simply removed with gentle traction. For optimal sensing and greater flexibility, closely spaced electrode pairs can be attached to the atrium and ventricle allowing the choice of unipolar or bipolar pacing modes. Waldo reported on the use of temporary epicardial wires in 70 consecutive patients undergoing cardiac surgery [31]. The ability to record an atrial electrogram assisted in diagnosing postoperative arrhythmias in 8 patients (11%). Therapeutic pacing was performed in 23 patients (33%) and the epicardial pacing leads were used for both purposes in an additional 26 patients (37%). Today, placement of temporary epicardial pacing leads has become the routine for most cardiac surgeries. These leads provide immediate therapy for a variety of bradycardias including heart block, and can be used to augment cardiac output by atrial overdrive pacing. They can also facilitate diagnosis of atrial or wide complex arrhythmias (by recording of intracardiac electrograms) and pacing termination of atrial flutter and other supraventricular tachycardias [31,32].

2.3. Can pacing therapy decrease the incidence of post-CABG AF?

In 1976, Waldo et al reported using temporary continuous rapid atrial pacing in two groups of post-cardiac surgery patients [33]. In the first group, recurrent episodes of severe hemodynamically compromising atrial flutter with 2:1 A:V block could be converted intentionally to AF which resulted in a slower ventricular rate or better rate control with pharmacological agents. Another group of postoperative patients suffered from recurrent episodes of paroxysmal atrial tachycardia, sustained ectopic atrial tachycardia, or sinus rhythm with premature atrial beats, that precipitated hemodynamically compromising AF. Continuous rapid atrial pacing resulted in 2:1 A:V block in all of these patients preventing SVT recurrence or AF.

Curiously, in the Multicenter Study of Perioperative Ischemia [8], an independent predictor of postoperative AF was postoperative atrial pacing (odds ratio 1.27). Atrioventricular pacing did not increase the likelihood of postoperative AF. As the response mode (demand or asynchronous) was not recorded, it was concluded that loss of AV synchrony may have been responsible for the higher incidence of AF, as is found in chronic pacing for sick sinus syndrome. The authors recommended AAI, or preferably DDD pacing, in patients requiring or using postoperative pacing.

The results of a randomized controlled trial of atrial overdrive pacing for the prevention of post-CABG AF were presented at the November 1996 American Heart Association annual meeting [34]. In this study, 100 post-CABG patients were randomized to AAI pacing at 10 beats per minute faster than the intrinsic heart rates or to no pacing therapy at all. Pacing was initiated within 24 hours of surgery and continued through postoperative day 4. AF occurred by postoperative day 4 in 13 of

51 (25.5%) of patients being paced and in 14 of 49 (28.6%) of control patients. The investigators concluded that, "contrary to common practice after CABG, atrial overdrive pacing in the AAI mode did not prevent postoperative AF." A concern raised by these investigators was the number of patients randomized to AAI pacing mode who could not be reliably paced in this mode primarily due to problems with atrial sensing. There was also a difference in use of beta-blocker therapy in the two groups, which could have influenced the AF incidence. This group of investigators, therefore, repeated this study using a pacemaker with enhanced sensing, automatic mode switching and consistent atrial overdrive pacing capabilities. The results of the Second Post Operative Pacing Study (POPS-2) were presented at the March 1998 meeting of the American College of Cardiology [35]. In this study, the temporary epicardial wires of 86 post-CABG patients were connected to a dual chamber rate responsive pacemaker. Patients were randomized to control or to be paced at a lower rate of 80 beats per minute with an upper rate of 130 beats per minute utilizing a programmed algorithm that maintained atrial overdrive pacing. Atrial fibrillation was seen in 11 of 43 (34%) of patients in both groups. An equal number of patients in both groups received beta-blockers thereby controlling for this previously confounding variable. The authors once again concluded that atrial overdrive pacing made no difference in the incidence of post-CABG AF.

2.4. Is there a future role for prophylactic pacing?

2.4.1. Studies of dual-site atrial pacing. Alessie [36] has suggested that both areas of conduction block and dispersion of atrial refractoriness may be critical in producing the multiple wavelets responsible for AF. Simultaneous biatrial or dual-site atrial pacing can eliminate dispersion of atrial refractoriness and prevent delayed atrial activation [36,37]. This may explain how atrial pacing, especially multiple site atrial pacing, may prevent recurrent AF.

Table 1.   Temporary postoperative pacing to prevent AF

Trial	Number of Patients	Mode of Pacing	Incidence of AF (%)	Comments
Chung[34]	49	None	28.6	NS
	51	AOO	25.5	
Schweiker[35]	43	None	34	Equal numbers were
	43	DDDR	34	taking BB
Mittelman[42]	62	None	35	
		AAI	29	NS
		Biatrial	33	
		None + BB	42	Paced vs. non-paced p=0.07
		AAI + BB	15	P=0.15
		Biatrial + BB	0	P=0.054
Orr[43]	78	None	27	P=0.13
		Biatrial (AAT)	18	
Goette[45]	37	RA (AAI)	53	
		Bachmann's Bundle	29	
Greenberg[44]	33	None + BB	31	Non-pacing (31%)
	31	RA + BB	10	compared to any mode
	29	LA + BB	17	of atrial pacing (13%)
	31	Biatrial + BB	13	p=0.04

NS = not statistically different
BB = beta-blockers
RA = right atrium
LA = left atrium
AAI = right atrial, single site demand pacing
AOO = overdrive atrial pacing
DDDR = rate responsive, AV sequential pacing
Biatrial (AAT) = simultaneous right and left atrial overdrive pacing

By pacing simultaneously from the right atrium as well as from within the coronary sinus, Daubert et al demonstrated that, at least in patients with severe interatrial conduction defects, biatrial pacing was associated with a low recurrence rate of AF and atrial flutter [38]. Saksena et al. have used a dual-site right atrial pacing system and tested its efficacy in preventing recurrent AF [39]. In this study, 15 patients with recurrent drug refractory AF and bradyarrhythmias requiring permanent pacing underwent implantation of a pacing system consisting of a standard right ventricular apical lead, an active fixation atrial lead placed at the os of the coronary sinus in the posterior right atrium, and another right atrial lead placed conventionally in the high right atrium. The atrial leads were connected to the atrial port of a DDDR pacemaker using a Y connector. This configuration allowed for both simultaneous unipolar dual-site right atrial pacing using the tip electrodes of both atrial leads as well as conventional atrial pacing from the high right atrium by simply programming the atrial output from bipolar to unipolar modes. Patients were placed in a dual-site-pacing mode for 3 months and subsequently mode switched to single site pacing for 3 months with subsequent mode switching every 6 months. With a mean follow-up of over 12 months, no AF recurrences were found in any patient during dual-site atrial pacing compared to 5 recurrences in 12 patients during single-site pacing (3 patients reported such great improvement in symptoms during the initial dual-site pacing mode that they refused to allow reprogramming to single-site pacing). The arrhythmia-free interval prior to pacing was 14 $\pm$ 14 days and increased to 89±7 days with dual-site pacing and to 76±27 with single-site pacing. Thus, at least in this small and nonrandomized study, the strategy of dual-site pacing was found to be both safe and at least as successful as conventional pacing modes in preventing AF. Additional studies by this group including a long-term comparison between single and dual site atrial pacing to prevent AF, support these conclusions [40,41].

2.4.2. Biatrial pacing modes to prevent post-CABG AF. Mittleman et al. presented preliminary data on post-CABG AF in patients treated with several different temporary pacing modes [42]. All 62 post-CABG patients had pairs of epicardial electrodes placed on the high lateral right atrium and the posteromedial left atrium in addition to ventricular electrodes. Patients were randomized to no pacing, AAI pacing or DDD pacing at 100 beats per minute using right atrial or biatrial pacing. They found 20 patients (32%) developed AF within 4 days of their surgery. There were no significant differences in AF incidence with the different pacing modes; there was a trend toward lower AF occurrence in patients on beta blockers. For patients on beta-blockers, the occurrence of AF in non-paced patients was 42% compared to 15% in patients paced only from the right atrium and 0% in patients paced simultaneously from the right and left atria.

The findings of a pilot study to assess the feasibility of synchronized biatrial pacing to prevent AF after CABG were recently presented at the March 1998 American College of Cardiology Annual Scientific Sessions [43]. In this effort, 78 patients undergoing CABG had epicardial electrodes placed on both the right and left atria. Patients were randomized to no pacing or biatrial pacing in the AAT mode ensuring synchronized atrial depolarization. The incidence of AF was

27% in the control patients and 18% in patients with biatrial pacing (p=0.13). The median duration of breakthrough episodes of AF was markedly less in patients with biatrial pacing (10 hrs. verses 48 hrs., p=0.035).

In a trial of atrial pacing in addition to beta-blocker therapy following CABG, three modes of pacing were compared for their ability to prevent postoperative AF [44]. Epicardial pacing wires were attached to both the right and left atria in 123 patients undergoing CABG. Patients were randomized to no pacing [33], right atrial pacing [31], left atrial pacing [29] or to biatrial pacing [31] for the first three days after surgery. All patients were also started on beta-blocker therapy as soon as they were extubated. The incidence of AF in the non-pacing group was 31% versus only 13% for patients randomized to one of the pacing strategies (p = 0.04; 95% CI 0.11-0.96). No significant difference between the tested pacing modes was seen with regard to AF incidence.

These very preliminary studies (Table 1) do not definitively support the notion of biatrial pacing to prevent AF, at least in the post-CABG patient. Additional study is needed to clarify ideal positioning of leads and the optimal mode of stimulation. Larger trials will be necessary to establish any benefit for subgroups or whether AF can be modified.

2.4.3. Bachmann's Bundle Pacing. Because both atrial sensing and capture thresholds are frequently unreliable when epicardial atrial temporary pacing wires are placed routinely (lateral right atrial wall), a study placing the atrial epicardial leads at the roof of the atria, into Bachmann's Bundles (a thick, muscular strand electrically connecting the right and left atria) was performed [45]. Sixty-three patients undergoing CABG were randomized to have atrial temporary pacing wires placed at the lateral wall (37 patients) or placed at Bachmann's Bundle (26 patients). All patients were overdrive paced (AAI) at 96 bpm for 4 days post CABG. The primary purpose of the study was to demonstrate a reliable alternative site for atrial pacing and, indeed, better sensing and capture were seen with Bachmann's Bundle pacing. An important additional observation, however, was a lower incidence of AF in those paced from Bachmann's Bundles, 29 %, compared to 53 % in patients paced at the lateral right atrium.

3. Role of Electrical Cardioversion

Direct current electrical cardioversion is clearly indicated in the patient who becomes hemodynamically compromised with post-CABG AF. Many clinicians prefer to routinely perform electrical cardioversion of AF in post-CABG patients to improve cardiac output by re-establishing AV synchrony. Patients are frequently uncomfortable in AF even with good ventricular rate control or may be intolerant of pharmacological therapies, suggesting another benefit from restoration of normal sinus rhythm by countershock. Conventional therapy is shock delivery via transthoracic paddles or adhesive pads.

The feasibility of using a new single lead catheter to perform internal cardioversion was recently reported [46]. Nine patients with AF after open heart surgery participated. A 7.5-F catheter (EP Medical, Berlin, NJ) was introduced via a brachial vein. When the catheter tip was in the right atrium, a balloon was inflated and with the aid of a guidewire, the catheter tip was advanced to the left pulmonary artery. The catheter had a distal electrode array (cathode, with 2.5 cm ^{2} surface) which thus positioned was near the left atrium, and a proximal array which was close to the lateral right atrial wall. An additional ring electrode was located midway between these arrays (in the right ventricle) and used for synchronized triggering. With the application of an R wave synchronized, biphasic 4±2 J shock, all patients were readily cardioverted with only minimal sedation. Three patients had an acute recurrence within 5 minutes, but 2 of these maintained sinus rhythms after an amiodarone bolus (150-mg IV) and a repeat shock. The advantage of this system would be the likely high success rates of cardioversion as well as the low energy requirements. The obvious disadvantages of performing cardioversion in this fashion is the need to perform an invasive procedure with risk of cardiac perforation (albeit very low), and the inability to perform the procedure rapidly in the event of hemodynamic compromise. It remains to be seen how this technique of cardioversion will be applied.

A system facilitating low energy internal cardioversion of AF utilizing prophylactically placed temporary epicardial wires has also been developed [TADpole, InControl, Redmond, WA 47,48]. These TADpole heart wires are very thin polyurethane-coated stainless steel wires comprised of 19 individual strands woven together for added strength and flexibility. They are sutured on to the epicardial surfaces of both atria in a manner similar to the placement of temporary epicardial pacing wires. In fact, these leads contain a 5-mm ring electrode that allows bipolar sensing and pacing as well as an 11.5-cm distal shocking electrode body. The right atrial wire is implanted encircling an area between the superior and inferior venae cavae and the left atrial wire is sutured onto the epicardial region between the AV groove and the left upper and lower pulmonary veins [Fig 1]. A third epicardial wire is secured to one of the ventricles to allow for R-wave synchronization. The wires are brought out through the skin and in the event of postoperative AF can be connected to an external defibrillator interface module, which in turn can be connected to a standard external defibrillator [Fig 2]. The interface unit attenuates the energy from the defibrillator by 97 % allowing for low energy, synchronized internal atrial defibrillation. In the largest report to date utilizing TADpole-heart wires [49], 100 consecutive patients undergoing open heart surgery had these special epicardial wires placed. AF occurred in 23 patients (23 %) at 2.1+/- 1.3 days postoperatively. In 16 of 20 patients (80 %), a synchronized shock of 5.2 +/-3 J terminated AF. Early recurrence (within 60 seconds) occurred in 8 patients. Five patients had multiple episodes of AF. A total of 35 episodes of AF were treated with a cardioversion success rate of 88 %. Of considerable clinical significance, only 6 patients (30 %) required any form of sedation. Over 530 patients have now had the TADpole- heart wires placed during open-heart surgery with over 100 episodes of spontaneous AF. Eighty-eight internal cardioversions have been attempted with an overall success rate of 53 % [personnel communication, InControl, Interim Data Report June 1998]. After each clinical center had performed 10 procedures, the success rate improved to 74 %, suggesting a learning curve phenomenon [50,51]. No difficulties with lead extraction or

126

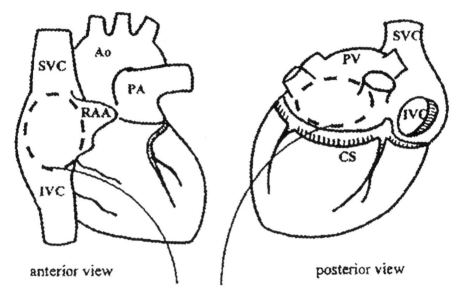

anterior view   posterior view

Figure 1. Two views of the human heart showing epicardial defibrillation wire electrodes in place. Distal 10 cm of wire is represented by an interrupted line forming an O-shaped surface area at right and left atria respectively. SVC = superior vena cava; IVC = inferior vena cava; RAA = right atrial appendage; Ao = aorta; PA = pulmonary artery; PV = pulmonary veins; CS = coronary sinus. (From: Liebold A, Wahba A and BirnbaumDE. Low energy cardioversion with epicardial wire electrodes. Reproduced with permission from The American Heart Association, Circulation 1998;98:883-886.)

complications with defibrillation have been encountered. In these preliminary studies, most patients did not request sedation even when they were scheduled for a repeat shock for recurrence of AF, and general anesthesia was not required for any patient.

This system appears to offer the advantages of safety, high efficacy and good tolerance. It performs low energy internal atrial cardioversion as well as atrial sensing for diagnostics and pacing, ventricular sensing and pacing, and AV sequential pacing. This system offers the potential for routine use in place of the typical simple temporary pacing wires in use today; further study is needed especially in regards to cost issues.

Figure 2. The TADpole system consists of epicardial leads sutured onto the heart during open heart surgery. These leads are brought out through the chest wall and

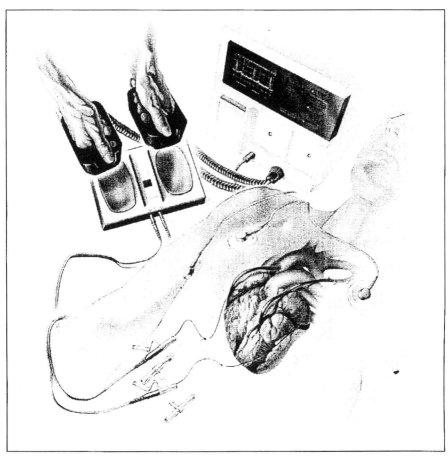

Illustration by K.E. Sweeney Illustration

can be attached to an interface unit that in turn can be connected to a standard external defibrillator. (see text for additional details)

128

4. Surgical Procedures for AF

In selected patients who have had disabling AF prior to surgery, additional surgical options are available.

The left atrium isolation procedure may restore a normal rhythm to the right atrium. This procedure was originally designed and applied to patients with refractory left atrial ectopic tachycardias [52], but has been used to treat AF as well [53]. In this procedure, a standard left atriotomy incision is extended anteriorly across Bachmann's Bundle to the level of the mitral valve annulus. It is further extended posteriorly to the coronary sinus as well as through the endocardium extending to the posterior aspect of the mitral valve annulus. Both the coronary sinus and the AV groove fat pad are dissected free of the atrium. A series of cryolesions are applied within the coronary sinus to disrupt any atrial fibers located in this region and the atriotomy is sutured closed [54]. This procedure was successfully applied by an Italian group to 100 patients with AF undergoing valvular surgery [53]. Over 80% of patients resumed sinus rhythm postoperatively. After 2 years follow-up, 70% of patients were able to maintain sinus rhythm. Of course, this procedure leaves the left atrium fibrillating or electrically silent and these patients must still be anticoagulated. However, chronotropic control was achieved and the restoration of right atrial transport was reported to improve overall left ventricular performance. According to the authors, one important additional advantage to this approach was the relative ease in performing the procedure with minimal additional ischemic time necessary for the isolation procedure's completion.

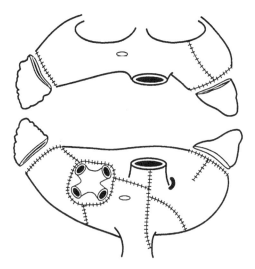

Figure 3. A schematic representation of the latest modification of the MAZE procedure: The atria are viewed anteriorly (above) and posteriorly (below). Both atrial appendages are removed and suture lines partition atrial tissue as shown. Note that the pulmonary vein orifices are isolated from the rest of the atrial tissue. (From: Cox JL. Evolving applications of the Maze procedure for atrial fibrillation. Reprinted with permission from The Society of Thoracic Surgeons, Annals of Thoracic Surgery 1993;55:578-580.)

The MAZE procedure pioneered by Cox [55-58], attempts to disrupt the multiple reentrant circuits found in both the right and left atria in patients with AF. By performing a series of cryolesions on both the epicardial and endocardial surfaces, reentrant circuits are prevented when there is insufficient distance between these lesions, fixed obstacles or non-conducting fibrous skeleton (i.e. reducing contiguous atrial tissue below the critical mass needed for AF) [56]. Following this procedure, at least theoretically, the only sustainable conduction pathway begins at the sinus node region, propagates anteriorly to the atrial septum, and down to the AV node. It continues across the septum to the left atrium where it is able to conduct from anterior to posterior beneath the pulmonary veins (see Fig 3).

Thus, both atria are able to depolarize sequentially and controlled input from the sinus node to the AV node is maintained. The results of 75 patients undergoing this procedure were reviewed in 1993 [59]. These patients had paroxysmal AF or atrial flutter (n=30) or chronic AF (n=36). Although normal AV synchrony was reestablished in all patients postoperatively, a rapid form of reentry atrial flutter was commonly seen but readily controlled with antiarrhythmic drug therapy. Only 1 spontaneous episode of AF was observed during a follow-up of more than 3 months, and 11% of patients required long term anticoagulation therapy for recurrent atrial flutter. Reestablishment of atrial transport was documented with intraoperative transesophageal echo and confirmed postoperatively with mitral and tricuspid color flow Doppler studies in all patients [60].

It has been proposed that the MAZE procedure may be appropriately performed in conjunction with valvular surgery [61], and it may be reasonable to consider in patients undergoing CABG, if a high enough risk population can be identified [62]. The MAZE procedure, unlike the left atrial isolation procedure, requires much more time on bypass and appears to result in a higher incidence of sinus node damage requiring pacemaker implant.

5. Conclusion

Following open heart surgery, AF continues to be a significant concern. Improvement in operative techniques has not reduced the incidence of postoperative AF. Even less invasive procedures such as the MIDCAB have not reduced AF incidence [63] but further work in this area continues. Temporary pacing, while certainly critical for hemodynamic support in some postoperative patients, has been disappointing as a preventive measure. New pacing modalities offer some promise and continue to be explored. Thus, it remains likely that for the foreseeable future, clinicians will need to continue dealing with AF after open heart surgery. New techniques of cardioversion may result in greater ease of restoration of sinus rhythm, and frequently may even obviate the need for sedation. Finally, we may see further evolution and utilization of surgical interventions, such as the MAZE procedure, to be performed in conjunction with CABG and valve surgeries in patients identified at the highest risk of developing chronic AF or its complications.

130

References

1. Langan MS and Horowitz LN. Cardiac surgery and cardiac trauma in current management of arrhythmia. 1991 Ed. Horowitz Decker, Inc. p 273.

2. lMichelson EL, Morganroth J, MacVaugh H III. Postoperative arrhythmias after coronary artery and cardiac valvular surgery detected by long-term electrocardiographic monitoring. Am Heart J 1979;97:442-8.

3. Rubin DA, Nieminski KE, Reed GE, Herman MV. Predictors, prevention and long-term prognosis of atrial fibrillation after coronary artery bypass graft operations. J. Thoracic Cardiovasc Surg 1987;94:331-5.

4. Laver MS, Eagle KA, Buckley MJ. DeSanctis RW. Atrial fibrillation following coronary artery bypass surgery. Prog Cardiovasc Dis 1989;31:367-78.

5. Crosby LJ, Pifalo WB, Woll KR, Burkholder JA. Risk factors for atrial fibrillation after coronary artery bypass grafting. Am J Cardiol 1990;66:1520-22.

6. Leitch JW, Thompson D, Baird DK, Harris PJ. The importance of age as a predictor of atrial fibrillation and flutter after coronary artery bypass grafting. J Thorac Cardiovasc Surg 1990;100:338-42.

7. Creswell LL, Shuessler RB, Rosenblum M, Cox JL. Hazards of postoperative atrial arrhythmias. Ann Thorac Surg 1993;56:539-49.

8. Mathew JP, Parks R, Savino JS, Friedman AS, Koch C, Mangano DT, Browner WS. Atrial fibrillation following coronary artery bypass graft surgery. JAMA 1996;276:300-6.

9. Paull DL, Tidwell SL, Guyton SW, Harvey E, Woolf RA, Holmes JR, Anderson RP. Beta blockade to prevent atrial dysrhythmias following coronary bypass surgery. Am J Surg 1997;173:419-21.

Fontan F, Madonna F, Naftel DC, Kirklin JW, Blackstone EH, Digerness S. Modifying myocardial management in cardiac surgery: a randomized trial. Eur J Cardiothorac Surg 1992;6:127-36.

11. Butler J, Chong JL, Rocker GM, Pillai R, Westaby S. Atrial fibrillation after coronary artery bypass grafting: a comparison of cardioplegia versus intermittent aortic cross-clamping. Eur J Cardiothorac Surg 1993;7:23-25.

12. The warm heart investigators. Randomized trial of hormothermic versus hypothermic coronary bypass surgery. Lancet 1994;343:559-63.

13. Daoud EG, Strickberger SA, Man KC, et al. Preoperative amiodarone as prophylaxis against atrial fibrillation after heart surgery. N Engl J Med 1997;337:1785-91.

14. Olshansky B. Post CABG IV amiodarone decreases incidence of atrial fibrillation - Results from ARCH. Am J Cardiol 1996;78:27-34.

15. Moss AJ, Rivers RJ, Cooper M. Long-term pervenous atrial pacing from the proximal portion of the coronary vein. JAMA 1969;209:543.

16. Davies JG, Sowton GE. Electrical threshold of the human heart. Br Heart J 196;28:231

17. Sutton R. Sinus node disease in clinical cardiac pacing [Ed Ellenbogen KA, Kay GN, Wilkoff BL] Saunders 1995; pp 284-303.

18. Sutton R, Kenny RA. The natural history of sick sinus syndrome. PACE 1986;9:1110-1114.

19. Rosenquist M, Brandt J, Schüler H. Long-term pacing in sinus node disease: effects of stimulation mode on cardiovascular morbidity and mortality. Am Heart J 19888;117:16-22.

20. Lamas GA, Estes NM III, Schneller S et al. Does dual-chamber or atrial pacing prevent atrial fibrillation? The need for a randomized controlled trial. PACE 1992;15:1109-1113.

21. Hesselson AB, Parsonnet V, Bernstein AD, Bonavita GJ. Deleterious effects of long-term single-chamber ventricular pacing in patients with sick sinus syndrome: the hidden benefits of dual-chamber pacing. J Am Coll Cardiol 1992;19:1542-1549.

22. Santini M, Alexidou G, Ansalone G, et al. Relation of prognosis in sick sinus syndrome to age, conduction defects and modes of permanent cardiac pacing. Am J Cardiol 1990;65:729

23. Anderson HR, Thuesen L, Bagger JP, Vesterlund T, Block Thomsen PE. Prospective randomized trial of atrial versus ventricular pacing in sick sinus syndrome. Lancet 1994;344:1523-1528.

24. Neilsen JC, Pedersen AK, Mortensen PT, Thuesen L, Vesterlund T, Block Thomsen PE et al. Atrial versus ventricular pacing in sick sinus syndrome. Long term follow-up in a prospective randomized trial of 225 consecutive patients [abstract] PACE 1997;20 (part II):1458.

25. Feuer JM, Shandling AH, Messenger JC, Castellanet CD, Thomas LA. Influence of cardiac pacing mode on long-term development of atrial fibrillation. Am J. Cardiol 1989;64:1376-1379.

26. Lamas GA. Pacemaker mode selection and survival: a plea to apply the principles of evidenced-based medicine to cardiac pacing practice. Heart 1997;78:218-20.

27. Charles RG, Mc Comb JM. Systematic trial of pacing to prevent atrial fibrillation (STOP-AF) Heart 1997;78: 224-225.

28. Zoll PM. Resuscitation of the heart in ventricular standstill by external electric stimulation. N Engl J Med 1952;247:768-71.

29. Shafiroff BGP, Linder J. Effects of external electrical pacemaker stimuli on the human heart. J Thorac Surg 1957;33:544-50.

30. Benson DW Jr, Dunnigan A, Benditt DG, Schneider SP. Transesophageal cardiac pacing: History, application, technique. Clin Prog Pacing Electrophysiol 1984;2:360-72.

31. Waldo AL, MacLean WAH, Cooper TB et al. Use of temporarily placed epicardial atrial wire electrodes for the diagnosis and treatment of cardiac arrhythmias following open heart surgery. J Thorac Cardiovasc Surg 1978;76:500-505.

32. Takeda M, Furuse A, Kotsuka Y. Use of temporary atrial pacing in management of patients after cardiac surgery. Cardiovasc Surg 1996;4:623-27.

33. Waldo AL, MacLean WA, Karp RB, Kouchoukos NT, James TN. Continuous rapid atrial pacing to control recurrent or sustained supraventricular tachycardias following open heart surgery. Circulation 1976;54:245-50.

34. Chung MK, Augostini RS, Asher CR et al. A randomized, controlled study of atrial overdrive pacing for the prevention of atrial fibrillation after coronary artery bypass surgery [abstract]. Circulation 1996;94 (Suppl I) I-190.

35. Schweikert RA, Grady TA, Gupta N, Augostini RS et al. Atrial pacing in the prevention of atrial fibrillation after cardiac surgery: Results of the second postoperative pacing study (POPS-2). [abstract] J Am Coll Cardiol. 1998;31 (SuppA):117A.

36. Allessie MA, Lammers WJEP, Bonke FM et al. Experimental evaluation of Moe's multiple wavelet hypothesis of atrial fibrillation. In ipes PP, Jalife J (ed): Cardiac electrophysiology and arrhythmias. Orlando FL, Grune & Stratton 1985, p275.

37. Yu W, Chen S, Tai C, Feng A, Chang M. Effects of different atrial pacing modes on atrial electrophysiology: implicating the mechanisms of biatrial pacing in prevention of atrial fibrillation. Circulation. 1997; 96:2992-2996.

38. Daubert C, Mabo P, Bender V. Arrhythmia prevention by permanent atrial resynchronization in advanced interatrial block. Eur Heart J 1990;11:237-42.

39. Saksena S, Prakash A, Hill M, Krol RB et al. Prevention of recurrent atrial fibrillation with chronic dual-site right atrial pacing. J Am Coll Cardiol 1996;28:687-94.

40. Prakash A, Saksena S, Hill M, Georgberidze I et al. Long-term results with dual and single atrial pacing for prevention of refractory atrial fibrillation [abstract]. Circulation 1996;94 Suppl I: I-68.

41. Prakash A, Saksena S, Kavshik R, Krol RB et al. Right and left atrial activation patterns during dual site right atrial pacing [abstract] PACE 1996;19:697.

42. Mittleman RS, Hill MRS, Mehra R, French SN et al. Evaluation of the effectiveness of righ atrial and biatrial pacing for the prevention of atrial fibrillation (AF) after coronary artery bypass surgery (CABG) [abstract]. Circulation 1996;94 Suppl I:I-68.

43. Orr WP, Tsui S, Stafford PJ, Pillai R, Bashir Y. Feasibility of synchronized bi-atrial pacing for preventing of atrial fibrillation after coronary artery bypass surgery - a pilot study [abstract]. J Am Coll Cardiol 1998;31:Suppl A 117A.

44. Greenberg MD, Katz NM, Tempesta BJ, et al.. Atrial pacing following cardiovascular surgery reduces the incidence of postoperative atrial fibrillation [abstract]. Circulation 1998;98: I: I-509.

45. Goette A, Mittag J, Friedl A, Busk H et al. Continuous pacing Bachmann's bundle after coronary artery bypass surgery [abstract] PACE 1998; Vol 21:April Part II p. 892.

46. Schneider MAE, Zrenner B, Karch MR, et al. Internal cardioversion of postoperatively occurring atrial fibrillation in patients undergoing cardiac surgery – first experiences using a new single lead catheter [abstract] PACE 1998; 21, Part II: 854.

47. Ortiz J, Sokolowski MC, Ayers GM, et al. Atrial defibrillation using temporary epicardial defibrillation stainless steel electrodes: studies in the canine sterile pericarditis model. J Am Coll Cardiol 1995; 26: 1356 – 1364.

48. Smolick BL, Ortiz J, Ayers GM, et al. Successful atrial defibrillation with very – low – energy shocks by means of temporary epicardial wire electrodes. J Thorac Cardiovasc Surg 1996; 111: 392 – 398.

49. Liebold A, Wahba A, Birnbaum DE. Low energy cardioversion with epicardial wire electrodes: new treatment of atrial fibrillation after open heart surgery. Circulation 1998; 98: 883 – 886.

132

50. Kleine P, Machner M, Nolte Th, Schäfer P, Laas J. Early versus late termination of atrial fibrillation following coronary artery bypass grafting using TADpole heart wires for internal defibrillation [abstract] PACE 1998; Vol 21:April, Part II p 952.

51. Kleine P, Blommaert D, van Nooten G, et al. Multicenter results of the Tadpole heartwire system used to treat postoperative atrial fibrillation [abstract]

52. Williams JM, Ungerleider GK, Lofland GK, Cox JL. Left atrial isolation. New Technique for the treatment of supraventricular arrhythmias. J Thorac Cardiovasc Surg 1980; 80: 373.

53. Graffigna A, Pagani F, Minzinoni G, et al. Left atrial isolation associated with mitral valve operations. Ann Thorac Surg 1992; 54: 1093 – 1098.

54. Cox JL. The surgical management of cardiac arrhythmias. In Sabaston DC, Jr., Spencer FC (eds.): Gibbon's Surgery of the Chest 4th ed. Philadelphia, WB Saunders, 1983 p 1566.

55. Ferguson TB, Jr. and Cox JL. Surgical treatment of cardiac arrhythmias. In Chatterjee K, Cheitlin MD, Karliner J, et al. (eds.): Cardiology an illustrated text/reference. Philadelphia, Lippincott/Gower, 1991 pp 6185 – 6214.

56. Cox JL, Boineau JP, Schuessler RB, et al. A review of surgery for atrial fibrillation. J Cardiac Electrophysiol 1991; 2: 541 – 561.

57. Cox Jl, Schuessler RB, D'Agostino HJ, et al. The surgical treatment of atrial fibrillation III. Development of a definitive surgical procedure. J Thorac Cardiovasc Surg 1991; 101: 569 – 583.

58. Cox JL. The surgical treatment of atrial fibrillation: IV surgical technique. J Thorac Cardiovasc Surg 1991; 101: 584 – 592.

59. Cox JL, Boineau JP, Schuessler RB et al. Five year experience with the MAZE procedure for atrial fibrillation. Ann   Thorac Surg 1993;56:814-24.

60. Hand DE, Lappas, Hogue CW, Cox JL. Perioperative transesophageal doppler echocardiographic verification of atrial transport function following the Maze procedure for atrial fibrillation. Surg Forum 1992; XLIII: 267 – 269.

61. McCarthy PM, Cosgrove DM, Castle LW, et al. Combined treatment of mitral regurgitation and atrial fibrillation with valvuloplasty and maze procedure. Am J Cardiol 1992; 72: 483 – 486.

62. Cox JL. Evolving applications of the Maze procedure for atrial fibrillation. Ann Thorac Surg 1993; 55: 578 – 580.

63. Tamis JE, Vloka ME, Malhotra S, Mindich BP and Steinberg JS. Atrial fibrillation is common after minimally invasive direct coronary artery bypass surgery. [absract] J AM Coll Cardiol 1998;31:118.

9 THERAPEUTIC OPTIONS FOR ESTABLISED OR RECURRENT ATRIAL FIBRILLATION: FOCUS ON ANTITHROMBOTIC THERAPY

John H. McAnulty, MD and Jack Kron, MD,
Oregon Health Sciences University,
Portland, OR

1. Introduction

A stroke at any time may be devastating. This is just as true after heart surgery. Recognized perioperative cerebrovascular accidents, with a permanent deficit, occur in approximately three percent of patients undergoing coronary artery bypass graft surgery. Another three percent develop seizures or deterioration of neurologic function [1-3] (Table 1). Following valve surgery, the rates of embolic events are slightly higher (with over 90% of the emboli involving the brain) [4-7] (Table 1). Emboli from manipulation of atherosclerotic aortas probably explain a majority of these neurologic events; [3] some may be due to thromboemboli.

Up to twenty-five percent of patients undergoing bypass graft surgery will have, or have had, atrial fibrillation [8]. Another five to forty percent will develop atrial fibrillation in the peri-operative period [1-10]. With the possible exception of "lone atrial fibrillation" (variably described as atrial fibrillation occurring intermittently in individuals under sixty years old who have no organic heart disease), atrial fibrillation is associated with an increased risk of stroke. On average, the stroke risk exceeds 5%/year in patients who are untreated [11-15]. Risk factors increasing the likelihood of stroke include: hypertension, reduced left ventricular function and a previous embolic event [16]. If an individual has none of these associated risk factors,

134

the risk of stroke per year may be as low as 2.5 %/year and an even lower 1.4%/year if the patient does not have diabetes [16].

Thus, in addition to the potential hemodynamic consequences of peri-operative atrial fibrillation with associated prolonged hospitalizations, the occurrence of this rhythm raises the concern of future strokes. The concern is appropriate but there is very little data to guide management as so little is known about the risk of stroke as it relates to this common, often transient, peri-operative event.

In most clinical situations, the following rule is probably applicable: "once an atrial fibrillation patient, always an atrial fibrillation patient". It is expressed to emphasize the point that, the risk of stroke is just as great in patients who are in sinus rhythm but who have had atrial fibrillation as it is in patients with continued atrial fibrillation [11-16]. Thus, the need to protect these individuals against a stroke is not dismissed by the presence of sinus rhythm. If this rule applies in the population of post operative patients who develop transient atrial fibrillation, the risk of a stroke approaches five percent per year. All need treatment.

If warfarin were the only effective available stroke preventive measure, it would be difficult to apply this rule to all postoperative patients. However, in most situations, aspirin, 325mg per day, is as protective against a stroke as warfarin in patients with atrial fibrillation [17,18,19]. Given this protective effect of aspirin, the recommendations of protecting patients against neurologic events following cardiac surgery becomes somewhat easier.

We recommend anti-thrombotic therapy in all post-op cardiac surgery patients. It is recognized this is somewhat controversial – an argument will be presented to convince the reader that the approach has some merit using the following clinical scenarios.

2. Clinical Scenarios and Recommendations Following Coronary artery bypass graft surgery

2.1. No recognized atrial fibrillation

It is important to note that the lack of recognition of atrial fibrillation does not mean it didn't occur. Patients may not be monitored and in some studies, patients were considered not to have had atrial fibrillation if a documented episode lasted less than five minutes. With the intention of minimizing the chance of a stroke it is recommended (by these authors) that all coronary graft surgery patients take aspirin, 325 mg per day. While lesser doses could be supported for the purpose of keeping grafts or vessels open, the argument to give 325 mg. is made because that has been the only dose that has been shown to prevent strokes in atrial fibrillation patients [17,19] and because the increased bleeding risk associated with it, compared to lower doses, is trivial. Thus, while aspirin may also be instituted for other purposes, it fortunately has a strong protective effect against neurologic events should the patient have had, or develop, atrial fibrillation.

2.2. Transient postoperative atrial fibrillation

It is not clear that these patients are at any different risk of a stroke than the just mentioned group that has not had atrial fibrillation. In one study, (with the length of follow-up not defined) a post-operative stroke rate of 3.7 percent was observed in patients who had transient atrial fibrillation compared to one percent in patients who did not have atrial fibrillation [1]. In other studies, atrial fibrillation was not associated with perioperative neurologic events [2,9]. For the same reasons given above, all patients should be treated with aspirin 325 mg./day. This is a life long recommendation. If a patient with transient post operative atrial fibrillation has risk factors that have been associated with a higher incidence of thromboembolic event in patients taking aspirin as compared to warfarin [17,20] (persistent uncontrolled hypertension with a systolic blood pressure greater than 160, severe LV dysfunction (somewhat arbitrarily defined as an EF <0.30), a history of a previous thromboembolic event), then consideration of the use of chronic warfarin therapy is appropriate, particularly if the patient can reliably and safely use this drug.

2.3. Persistent postoperative atrial fibrillation (continuous or intermittent)

 Stroke prevention treatment should be the same as with any other patient with chronic atrial fibrillation. In many cases the aspirin 325 mg. would be adequate unless the patient has one of the risk factors for thromboemboli [15,20].

2.4. The patient who had known preoperative atrial fibrillation

Decisions about chronic stroke prevention treatment in the patient already known to have atrial fibrillation should not be influenced by the surgery (except for the transient withholding of therapy for the surgery itself) [11-15,17,19,20].

3. Valve Surgery

3.1. Mechanical valves

Patients receiving these valves require immediate post-operative anti-thrombotic therapy and chronic anti-coagulation therapy with warfarin. The effect of peri-operative atrial fibrillation on the incidence of thromboembolic events is not clear but it becomes less relevant given the fact that the anti-coagulation is required even unrelated to the rhythm (Table 3) [21].

3.2. Tissue valves

There is little information about the significance of peri-operative atrial fibrillation as it relates to the incidence of thromboembolic events in patients receiving a tissue valve. In one large series evaluating the risk of thromboemboli after tissue valve replacement, atrial fibrillation was specifically evaluated as a risk factor and was found not to contribute to the incidence of subsequent thromboembolic events [4].

If a patient receives a tissue mitral valve, it is currently recommended – in part because of the concerns of an increased incidence of atrial fibrillation with the valve in this position – that anti-thrombotic therapy with heparin and then warfarin should be started early after the prosthesis is inserted and that it should be continued for at least three months [4]. In the patient who has chronic atrial fibrillation or has had fibrillation unrelated to the surgery, long-term warfarin therapy is required. It's not clear if transient perioperative atrial fibrillation is a reason to continue long-term warfarin therapy, but if a patient is a good warfarin candidate, that recommendation is reasonable. If not a good warfarin candidate, aspirin (325 mg/day) would seem appropriate.

There is debate about the need for anti-thrombotic therapy following insertion of a tissue valve in the aortic position. The early high risk of perioperative embolic strokes has led some to recommend early postoperative treatment with heparin and warfarin [4]. Perioperative atrial fibrillation was found in 14% of those receiving an aortic prosthesis. It was not an independent predictor of a subsequent stroke [4]. Others found the 7.4% incidence of cerebral ischemic events at four months in those on anticoagulants to be no different from the 6.5% incidence in those not treated with anticoagulants [7]. They did not relate these events to the observed 20% incidence of atrial fibrillation. Neither study was prospective or randomized. The presence of peri-operative atrial fibrillation would strengthen the argument for at least the three-month use of warfarin and long-term use of aspirin therapy.

4. Congenital Heart Surgery

The role of peri-operative atrial fibrillation as it relates to subsequent thromboembolic events with congenital heart surgery is undefined. Until more is known, aspirin would be reasonable therapy for at least a few months in patients with atrial arrhythmias with the consideration of the need for a long-term therapy depending on other thromboembolic risk factors. The presence of significant risk factors would be a reason to consider long-term warfarin therapy, again, somewhat unrelated to the peri-operative nature of the atrial fibrillation.

4.1. Diagnostic studies and newer antithrombotic treatment for perioperative atrial fibrillation

In this 1999 chapter, at least a consideration of newer diagnostic and treatment modalities seems necessary. It is only because they are left out up to this point that they are now mentioned because they don't clearly contribute in a major way to directing stroke prevention therapy for perioperative atrial fibrillation. In one study [22], left atrial size as determined by transthoracic echocardiography was useful in predicting a higher stroke risk in patients with nonvalvular atrial fibrillation. Thus, if found in any of the patients depicted in the previous scenarios, left atrial enlargement would be more of a reason to support chronic antithrombotic therapy; it hasn't been shown to determine those better treated with aspirin versus warfarin.

Transesophageal echocardiography may be useful in directing therapy in individual cases. The higher association of ulcerated plaques with strokes in other patients with atrial fibrillation [23] suggests that transesophageal echocardiography might be considered before all heart surgery, but it's role in broadly directing treatment choices in relation to perioperative atrial fibrillation is unclear.

Alternative antithrombotic agents such as the blockers of ADP induced platelet aggregation and the IIB, IIIA glycoprotein platelet receptor site blockers may be optimal in some patients but again, their role in treatment of perioperative (or chronic) atrial fibrillation are not defined.

Table 1

Risk of Perioperative Neurologic Event*		
Heart Surgery	Neurologic Event	Relation to Atrial Fibrillation
CABG[1-3]	CVA 3% Neurologic Deficit 3%	Perioperative atrial fibrillation increased CVA risk in one study[1] but not in others [2,9]
Valve Surgery [4-7] Mechanical** Aortic Mitral		Not defined
Tissue*** Aortic Mitral	6-7% 5-10%	No association recognized when evaluated
Congenital Defects Repair	5%	Not defined

* Perioperative – generally defined as out to 30 day
** with initiation of warfarin (and often early heparin)
*** without antithrombotic therapy

Table 2

Antithrombotic Therapy for Patients Who Have Perioperative Atrial fibrillation At the time of Coronary Artery Bypass Graft Surgery		
Rhythm Status	Post Op Rx	Chronic Treatment
No recognized atrial fibrillation	ASA, 325 mg QD	ASA, 325 mg QD
Transient post-op atrial fibrillation	ASA, 325 mg QD	ASA, 325 mg QD
Preoperative atrial fibrillation	ASA, 25 mg QD Or warfarin (INR 2-3)	ASA, 325 mg QD or warfarin (INR –3)
Post operative chronic atrial fibrillation	ASA, 325 mg QD Or warfarin (INR 2-3)	ASA, 325 mg QD Or warfarin (INR 2-3)

Table 3

Antithrombotic Therapy[a]– Prosthetic Heart Valves

	Mechanical Prosthetic Valves			Biological Prosthetic Valves		
	Warfarin INR 2-3	Warfarin INR 2.5-3.5	Aspirin 50-100 Mg	Warfarin INR 2-3	Warfarin INR 2.5-3.5	Aspirin 50-100 mg
First 3 months after valve replacement		+	+		+	+
After first 3 months						
Aortic Valve	+		+			+
Aortic valve + risk factor		+	+	+		+
Mitral valve		+	+			+
Mitral valve + risk factor		+	+		+	+

a Depending on the clinical status of patient, antithrombotic therapy must be individualized
b Risk Factors – atrial fibrillation, previous thromboembolus, LV dysfunction, hypercoagulable state [16]. Modified table used with permission [20].

References

1. Aranki SF, Shaw DP, Adams DH, Rizzo RJ, Couper GS. Predictors of atrial fibrillation after coronary artery surgery: current trends and impact on hospital resources. Circulation 1996;94:390-397.
2. Newman, MF, Wolman R, Kanchuger M, Marschall K, Mora-Mangano C. Multicenter preoperative stroke risk index for patients undergoing coronary artery bypass graft surgery. American Heart Association, Inc. 1996; II-74-II-80.
3. Roach GW, Kanchuger M, Mangano CM, Newman M, Nussmeier N, et al. Adverse cerebral outcomes after coronary bypass surgery. N Eng J Med 1996;335:1857-1863.
4. Heras M, Chesebro JH, Fuster V, Penny W, Grill D. High risk of thromboemboli early after bioprosthetic cardiac valve replacement. JACC 1995;11:1111-1119.
5. Davis EA, Greene PS, Cameron DE, Gott VL, Laschinger JC. Bioprosthetic versus mechanical prostheses for aortic valve replacement in the elderly. Circulation 1996;94:II-121-II-125.
6. Borger MA, Ivanov J, Weisel RD, Peniston CM, Mickleborough LL. Decreasing incidence of stroke during valvular surgery. Circulation 1998; II-137-II-143.
7. Moinudden K, Quin J, Shaw R, Dewar M, Tellides G. Anticoagulation is unnecessary after biological aortic valve replacement. Circulation 1998; II-95-II-99.
8. Mathew JP, Parks R, Savino JS, Friedman AS, Koch C, et al. Atrial fibrillation following coronary artery bypass graft surgery: predictors, outcomes, and resource utilization. JAMA 1996;276:1719-1720.
9. Lauer MS, Eagle KA, Buckley MJ, DeSanctis RW. Atrial fibrillation following coronary artery bypass surgery. Prog Cardiovasc Dis 1989;31:367-378.
10. Daoud EG, Strickberger SA, Man KC, Goyal R, Deeb GM, et.al. Preoperative amiodarone as prophylaxis against atrial fibrillation after heart surgery. New Eng J Med 1997;337:1785-1791.
11. Stroke Prevention in Atrial Fibrillation Investigators. SPAF Study final results. Circulation 1991;84:527-539.
12. Petersen P, Boysen G, Godtfredsen J, Andersen E, Andersen B. Placebo-controlled, randomised trial of warfarin and aspirin for prevention of thromboembolic complications in chronic atrial fibrillation: the Copenhagen study. Lancet 1989;1:175-178.
13. The Boston Area Anticoagulation Trial for Atrial Fibrillation Investigators. The effect of low-dose warfarin on the risk of stroke in patients with nonrheumatic atrial fibrillation. N Engl J Med 1990;323:1505.
14. Veterans Affairs Stroke Prevention in Nonrheumatic Atrial Fibrillation Investigators: Warfarin in the prevention of stroke associated with nonrheumatic atrial fibrillation. N Eng J Med 1992;327:1406-12.
15. Connolly SJ, Laupacis A, Gent M, et al. Canadian Atrial Fibrillation Anticoagulation (CAFA) Study. J Am Coll Cardiol 1991;18:349.
16. Stoke Prevention in Atrial Fibrillation Investigators. Predictors of thromboembolism in atrial fibrillation:1. Clinical features of patients at risk. Ann Intern med 1992;116:1-5.

17. Stroke Prevention in Atrial Fibrillation Investigators. Warfarin vs. aspirin for prevention of thromboembolism in atrial fibrillation: Stroke Prevention in atrial Fibrillation II Study. Lancet 1994;343:687-691.

18. Atrial Fibrillaton Investigators. Risk factors for stroke and efficacy of antithrombotic therapy in atrial fibrillation: analysis of pooled data from five randomized clinical trials. Arch Int med 1994;54:1949-1957.

19. Stroke Prevention in Atrial Fibrillation Investigators. Prospective identification of patients with nonvalvular atrial fibrillation at low-risk of stroke during treatment with aspirin. JAMA 1998;279:1273-77.

20. Stroke Prevention in Atrial Fibrillation Investigators. Adjusted-dose warfarin vs. low-intensidy, fixed-dose warfarin plus aspirin for high-risk patients with atrial fibrillation: Stroke prevention in Atrial Fibrillation III Study. Lancet 1996;348:633-638.

21. McAnulty JH, Rahimtoola SH. Antithrombotic therapy and valvular heart disease. In *Hurst's The Heart, 9th Edition*, Alexander R, Schlant R, Fuster V, ed. : McGraw-Hill Companies, Inc. 1998.

22. Stroke Prevention in Atrial Ribrillation Investigators. Predictors of thromboembolism in atrial fibrillation:II. Echocardiographic features of patients at risk. Annals Int med 1992;116:6-12

23. Zabalgoitia M, halperin JL, Pearce LA, Blackshear JL, Asinger RW, hart RG. Transesophageal echocardiographic correlates of clinical risk of thromboembolism in nonvalvular atrial fibrillation. J Am Coll Cardio 1998;31:1622-6.

10 ATRIAL FIBRILLATION AFTER NONCARDIAC SURGERY

Dhiraj D. Narula, MD and Jonathan S. Steinberg, MD,
St. Luke's-Roosevelt Hospital Center and
Columbia University College of Physicians and
Surgeons, New York, NY

1. Introduction

New onset atrial fibrillation is very common after cardiac surgery and though it occurs less frequently after other types of surgery, it is still a major clinical problem. With the large numbers of surgical procedures performed each year in the United States, even a small incidence translates into a significant absolute number of patients.

Thoracic noncardiac surgery, especially with lung resection, is associated with an impressive incidence of postoperative atrial fibrillation, up to 42%, higher than non-thoracic surgery. Abdominal and vascular surgery also have a measurable incidence of postoperative atrial fibrillation [1]. Despite improvements in anesthetics and monitoring techniques in the last decade, the incidence of cardiac arrhythmias remains high [2]; this may reflect in part an aging surgical population. The majority of published reports reflect observations on thoracic non-cardiac surgery; this will be the major focus of this chapter.

2. Atrial Fibrillation after Thoracic Noncardiac Surgery

2.1 Incidence

Table 1 lists published studies on the incidence of arrhythmias following thoracic surgery; the reported incidence varies from 1 to 42 %. Comparison of surgical series

STUDIES (TABLE 1)

YEAR	AUTHOR	N	SURGERY	ARRHYTHMIA DEFINITION	% ARR	% AF	COMMENT
1943	Currens[3]	56	thoracic	AF, AFL	21	14	
1943	Bailey[4]	78	lung (P)	SVA	12	8	
1946	Massie[5]	120	lung (P)	SVA, APC, VPC	9	4	only symptomatic arrhythmia
1955	Krosnick[6]	82	thoracic	SVA > 150 bpm	12	10	age > 50 y
1957	Cohen[7]	92	thoracic	SVA, APCs	16	8	
1957	Cerney[8]	76	lung	SVA, APC	21	14	
1958	Epstein[9]	286	lung$	SVA	21	16*	
1958	Hurt[10]	51@	lung$	AF, AFL	31	31*	
1960	Shields[11]	121	lung	AF, AFL, PAC, PVC	16	12*	age > 55 y
1961	Wheat[12]	302@	thoracic	SVA	17	16*	age > 55y
1961	Catalayud[13]	338	thoracic	SVA, APC, VPC, VT, AVB	4	1	chart review
1964	Mowry[14]	574	lung	SVA, SB, ST	4	3	
1967	Bergh[15]	81@	lung	AF	-	20	
1968	Shields[16]	50@	lung$	AF, AFL	14	14*	ecg q2d + prn
1969	Juler[17]	563	thoracic	SVA, VT, VPC	6	4	review
1969	Stougard[18]	260	lung (P)$	SVA, APC, VPC, VT	37	18	
1971	Ghosh[19]	100	thoracic	SVA, APC	34	16	ecg qd + prn
1972	Burman[20]	207	thoracic	SVA, PVC, VT	6	-	age > 40 y monitored > 24 h
1973	Beck-Neilsen[21]	300	thoracic	SVA, ST, APC	21	13	ecg on d1, d3 + prn
1975	Alstrup[22]	60	lung$	AF	-	42	monitored 4d
1979	Adebo[23]	40 @	lung (P)	Unspecified	45	-	
1982	Nagasaki[24]	961	lung$	AF, AFL	4	4*	review
1982	Keagy[25]	90	lung (P)	SVA, APC, VPC	41	22*	
1984	Keagy[26]	43	lung	AF, AFL	7	7*	age > 70 y
1987	Krowka[27]	236	lung	SVA	22	14	"most" pts monitored
1988	Mathisen[28]	104	esophagus	AF	-	9	review, all given digitalis
1988	Schwarz[29]	89	scopy	AF	-	2	
1989	Wahi[30]	197	lung (P)	AF	-	23	review
1990	Ritchie[31]	140	thoracic	SVA, VT, VPC	37	18	monitored 4 d
1991	Von Knorring[2]	598	lung$	SVA	16	14	monitored 2-3 d
1993	Asamura[32]	267	thoracic	SVA, APC, VPC, brady	24	12	monitor in ICU + prn
1994	Van Meighem[33]	552	lung	AF	-	19	
1994	McDonald[34]	60	lung	AF	-	2	resection of breast cancer metastases
1995	Amar[35]	100	lung	SVA	18	16	symptoms or ecg
1996	Van Meighem[36]	99@	lung	AF	-	15	monitored 3d
1996	Allen[37]	771	scopy	AF	-	1	3% if converted to thoracotomy
1996	Terzi[38]	105@	thoracic	SVA	27	23	monitor 1-2d
1996	Swanson[39]	46	scopy	AF	-	11	
1997	Jakobsen[40]	15 @	lung	AF > 30 sec	-	40	monitored 4 d, ecg tid x 10 d

% ARR=percentage of patients who developed postoperative arrhythmia, %AF= percentage of patients who developed postoperative atrial fibrillation, scopy=thoracoscopy, AF=atrial fibrillation, AFL=atrial flutter, SVA=all supraventricular arrhythmias (including AF or AFL, atrial tachycardia, nodal tachycardia, supraventricular tachycardia) but not premature beats, APC=atrial premature beats, VPC=ventricular premature beats, VT=ventricular tachyarrhythmias (may include cardiac arrest), AVB=atrioventricular block, brady=bradyarrhythmias, @=placebo or control arm, $=only lung cancer, (P)=only pneumonectomy, *=includes AFL, h=hour, d=day, ecg prn=electrocardiogram recorded as per clinical need, ICU=intensive care unit is rendered difficult by varying definitions: studies include atrial fibrillation, atrial flutter and nonspecific supraventricular tachycardia; some even include atrial premature beats, ventricular premature beats, ventricular tachycardia or sinus tachycardia in the analysis. Atrial fibrillation comprises the majority of the reported arrhythmias, and its incidence is separately listed, if available from the original paper. The method and period of monitoring can impact on the reported incidence of arrhythmia, as can the choice of only clinically relevant episodes as opposed to asymptomatic ECG findings; these are also listed if available. The type and mix of surgery can also affect the incidence of atrial fibrillation; these differences may provide clues to the relative importance of putative mechanisms.

At first glance, the numbers seem highly inconsistent, as is expected given the various types of surgery and definitions of arrhythmia. The highest incidence of post-operative atrial fibrillation, greater than 40%, is reported in two small studies [22,40] of lung resection, with a generous definition of atrial fibrillation (>30 seconds) in one, and postoperative continuous monitoring for 4 days in both. The lowest are reported in studies [13,17,24] which relied solely on a retrospective chart review. Operative series involving esophagus surgery [28] or thoracoscopy [29,37] show a substantially lower incidence of postoperative atrial fibrillation. Studies that include other supraventricular tachyarrhythmias or even premature beats tend to demonstrate higher overall arrhythmia rates. Analysis of the 33 reports of lung or thoracic surgery with data on incidence of atrial fibrillation from Table 1 reveals that the median rate of atrial fibrillation from these studies was 14%. These 33 studies reported a total of 7053 patients and 810 (12%) developed postoperative atrial fibrillation.

3. Risk Factors Which Affect the Incidence of Atrial Fibrillation

3.1. Age

Atrial fibrillation is clearly a disease of the elderly; for each advancing decade of age the odds ratio for development of atrial fibrillation is 2.1 in men and 2.2 in women [41]. .In studies of atrial fibrillation following cardiac surgery, age emerges as a potent risk factor [42-45] . It is logical that the elderly should therefore be at a relatively greater risk for atrial fibrillation following thoracic surgery.

Several authors [9,14] have made this observation. Von Knorring [2] noted that 24% of patients aged 70 or more developed an arrhythmia as compared to 14% of those aged less than 70 years (p<0.05). Massie et al [5] noted that the incidence of cardiac arrhythmias was 9% overall, 14% in patients over 35 years of age and 22% in those aged over 60 years. In an analysis of risk factors for arrhythmias post-thoracic surgery, Asamuara [32] found that age remained a significant predictor (p<0.0001) in a multivariate model; arrhythmias occurred in 3% of patients aged <50 years, 25% of patients aged 50-69 years, and 50% of patients aged 70 years or more. Krosnick [6] noted that patients who developed arrhythmia had a mean age of 66 years as opposed to a mean age of 61 years in those who did not develop arrhythmia. Similarly, in Shields' series [16], patients who developed atrial fibrillation were, on average, 3 years older than those who did not. In some reports, atrial fibrillation was practically confined to those over 50 [7,8] or over 60 [16].

Dissenting voices are few. One small series of 43 patients [26] suggested a low 7% incidence of postoperative atrial fibrillation in patients over 70 years of age undergoing pulmonary resection.

Clearly, the elderly constitute a population at higher risk for development of postoperative atrial fibrillation. The magnitude of the problem in this group can be appreciated from the fact that more than 600,000 individuals 65 years of age or older require major abdominal or noncardiac surgery each year [46].

3.2. Extent of pulmonary resection/lymph node resection/type of surgery

3.2.1. Extent of Lung Resection. Several authors have observed a relation between the amount of lung tissue removed and the incidence of postoperative arrhythmias, particularly atrial fibrillation. Cerney [8] found that the incidence of supraventricular arrhythmia was approximately two-fold greater for pneumonectomy (29%) than for lobectomy (14%). In a study of 574 patients, Mowry [14] observed that arrhythmias documented by electrocardiograms occurred in 19% of patients after pneumonectomy, 3% after lobectomy and less than 1% after a segmental or wedge resection. In a series of patients with lung malignancy, Epstein [9] reported that the incidence of arrhythmias was 26% following pneumonectomy, 16% following lobectomy and 3% following thoracotomy without lung resection. Other authors [4,33] have also observed this relationship. Even in a series [21] that concluded that there was no relation between the extent of lung resection and the incidence of atrial fibrillation, the reported incidence was 22% with pneumonectomy, 20% with lobectomy and 16% with minor procedures including exploratory thoracotomy.

Breyer [47] observed postoperative atrial fibrillation in 13% following pneumonectomy and 5% after segmental or subsegmental resection. In this series, the risk of death was also related to the extent of pulmonary resection (odds ratio 2.8 for lobectomy or pneumonectomy versus segmental or subsegmental resection, p=0.017). Asamura [32] studied 267 operations for predictors of postoperative atrial fibrillation using a multivariate model. The incidence of arrhythmias increased stepwise (Figure 1) with the extent of pulmonary resection and remained a significant (p=0.0008) predictor in a multivariate analysis.

Procedures other than major lung resection have a lower risk. Von Knorring [2] found that 12% of 398 patients who underwent procedures other than pneumonectomy for lung malignancy developed arrhythmia, while 23% of 200 patients who underwent pneumonectomy (p<0.01) did. The patient population may impact on the reported incidence: McDonald [34] found that in a series of women of median age 58 years who underwent pulmonary wedge resection for metastatic breast cancer, only 1 of 60 developed atrial fibrillation.

The possible reasons for this are many. A more extensive dissection may cause a greater damage to the cardiac nerves and plexi; this may affect the autonomic control of the heart and affect the duration or the dispersion of atrial refractoriness [32]. A greater resection may result in higher pulmonary vascular resistance, both by anatomic reduction of the pulmonary vascular bed and increased

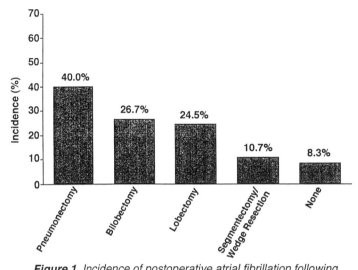

Figure 1. Incidence of postoperative atrial fibrillation following varying extent of lung resection.
From Asamura et al, J Thorac Cardiovasc Surg 1993; 1066; 1101-1110.

hypoxic pulmonary vasoconstriction. This, in turn, may result in an increase in right ventricular systolic and filling pressures, and increased right atrial stretch. A lesser residual lung area may result in lower pulmonary reserve and more hypoxia; a lower oxygen saturation may result in an increased susceptibility of the heart to arrhythmias [48].
.

3.2.2. Extent of lymph node resection. The extent of lymph node resection may affect the incidence of postoperative atrial fibrillation by increasing the extent of damage to the cardiac nerves and therefore autonomic control of the heart. In this regard, Cohen [7] found in a study of 92 patients who underwent thoracotomy that atrial arrhythmias were more frequent in patients who had mediastinal dissection. Asamura [32], in a study of 267 operations, found that the incidence of arrhythmias increased stepwise with the extent of lymph node dissection; however, this did not remain statistically significant in a multivariate analysis.

3.2.3. Pericardial incision. Incision of the pericardium may be necessary to allow complete tumor resection, remove metastases, or allow intrapericardial ligation of the pulmonary veins. Several experimental models of atrial fibrillation use sterile pericarditis [49,50]. Thus invasion of the pericardium may reasonably be expected to increase the incidence of atrial fibrillation after surgery. However, the data does not substantially support this hypothesis, and its role must therefore be presumed to be small.

Krowka [27], in a study of 236 patients who underwent pneumonectomy, found that tachydysrhythmias were more common in patients who had intrapericardial dissection; 53% vs. 7% (p<0.001). Hurt and Bates [10] reported that 45% of patients who underwent an intrapericardial resection developed atrial fibrillation or flutter after surgery as compared to 20% of patients who had an extrapericardial resection. On the other hand, Wahi [30], Beck-Neilsen [21], Epstein [9] and Adebo [23] reported no difference in the incidence of arrhythmias between patients who underwent pericardial incision and those who did not.

3.2.4. Minimally invasive thoracic procedures. Though no head to head comparison of incidence of atrial fibrillation after minimally invasive and conventional thoracic procedures has been reported, review of surgical series suggests that the incidence of atrial fibrillation is lower after minimally invasive procedures.

In a series of operative thoracoscopic procedures for the treatment of thoracic metastases [29], only 2 of 89 patients had postoperative atrial fibrillation. Lung volume reduction by the same route may add risk; in another series of thoracoscopic lung plication [39], atrial fibrillation occurred after 5 of 46 procedures and in a small series of thoracoscopic pneumonectomy [51], 1 of 6 patients had postoperative atrial fibrillation. In a series of patients who had video-assisted thoracoscopic surgery [37] , atrial fibrillation occurred in 1% of patients who had a closed procedure as opposed to 3% of those who required conversion to thoracotomy.

3.3. Right vs left pneumonectomy

Various studies have compared the incidence of arrhythmias after right or left pneumonectomy, and found varying results. Several authors [8,12,21] have found a higher incidence of arrhythmia and cardiac complications after right pneumonectomy; others [14,30,52] have found a higher incidence of arrhythmia after left sided surgery. In all these reports, except one [14], the differences are modest and either were not analyzed for or did not reach statistical significance. In the absence of a convincing biological hypothesis to explain either, the results, in our view, must be viewed as chance findings.

3.4. Underlying lung disease (malignant vs benign)

Beck-Neilsen [21] , in a series of 300 thoracotomies, noted atrial fibrillation in 20% (33 of 168) of patients with lung cancer as compared to 3% (2 of 64) patients with benign lung disease (p<0.001); the incidence was particularly low in patients who underwent thoracotomy for diseases of the esophagus or diaphragm. The extent of surgery was greater in patients with pulmonary malignancy; hence the authors made a comparison for minor resections and exploratory surgery; the difference was still significant (p<0.05) for a higher incidence of atrial fibrillation in patients with lung cancer (8 of 50) than benign disease (2 of 64). Patients with cancer were on average 2 years older than those with benign disease; this was not adjusted for and may in part explain the result.

The same group went on to investigate the hypothesis that lipolysis or other metabolic abnormalities might be correlated with and be causal for the onset of atrial fibrillation in patients with lung cancer undergoing thoracotomy. Alstrup and Sorensen [22] reported that 60 patients were evaluated; no difference was seen in serial glucose, serum insulin, glycerol and triglycerides, though serum free fatty acids rose at the onset of atrial fibrillation. The authors concluded that there was no evidence to suggest that a compromised intracellular mechanism in cancer might be responsible for the arrhythmia.

3.5. Preexisting cardiac disease

Preexisting cardiac disease does not seem to be a requisite for the development of atrial fibrillation, however since atrial fibrillation is generally more common in patients with heart disease, it is reasonable to suppose that this relationship should persist in the post-operative setting. The data supporting this premise is reasonably convincing.

Von Knorring [2] found the incidence of arrhythmia to be significantly higher in patients with remote myocardial infarction (26% vs 15%, p<0.05), in patients with congestive heart failure (30% vs 15%, p<0.05), in patients with ischemic changes on ECG (p<0.01) or an ischemic response to an exercise test (34% vs 14%, p<0.01) and in patients with arterial hypertension (26% vs 14%, p<0.05). Mowry [14] retrospectively identified 35 of their 574 patients as having cardiovascular disease; 26% developed arrhythmia as opposed to 2% of the others. On the other hand, Ritchie [31] found the incidence of postoperative arrhythmia to have no relation to preexisting myocardial disease (32% vs 38%, p>0.5) and Massie [5] reported that only 4% of patients with prior heart disease on clinical examination or electrocardiogram developed a postoperative arrhythmia while 11% of patients without heart disease did so.

Electrocardiographic predictors are more controversial. Shields concluded in one study [11] that a history of a prior arrhythmia or the presence of frequent premature ventricular beats appeared to be the only significant features that presage occurrence of postoperative atrial fibrillation or flutter. In another report [16] he noted, in addition, the presence of premature atrial contractions or a right bundle branch block as relevant. Epstein [9] concluded that a history of paroxysmal tachycardia, clinical evidence of multiple extrasystoles, or a left bundle branch block on the preoperative ECG appeared to be important. Many studies excluded patients with prior arrhythmias; it is reasonable to assume that postoperative arrhythmias may be more frequent in these cases. On the other hand, Wheat [12] felt that electrocardiograms did not help predict development of arrhythmias and Asamura [32] found that a preoperative electrocardiographic abnormality correlated with arrhythmia post-thoracic surgery only on a univariate analysis, but not on a multivariate analysis.

3.6. Infection/inflammation

Many authors have commented on the correlation of infection or inflammation and the occurrence of post-operative atrial fibrillation. Bailey [4] suggested in 1943 that infection of the pulmonary stump might be relevant in the genesis of atrial fibrillation. Cerney et al [8] noted that many of the patients in their series with postoperative atrial fibrillation had empyema or pneumonia evident almost simultaneously. Epstein [9] reported that pulmonary infection, bronchospasm, lung collapse and pulmonary embolism were the most frequent complications associated with postoperative arrhythmias. Cohen [7] , on the other hand, found no correlation between the occurrence of atrial arrhythmias and pulmonary infection prior to surgery or with postoperative fever. It is well recognized that in other clinical settings, for example, pneumonia in the elderly, atrial fibrillation may be precipitated by various stressors; thus it is not unreasonable to posit that there may be such a correlation in the postoperative setting. Clearly, though, causality is unproved, and the association is modest.

3.7. Postoperative volume overload

Krowka et al [27] reported that AF occurred more frequently in patients who developed post-operative interstitial pulmonary edema or perihilar pulmonary infiltrates (52% vs. 12%, p<0.001) following pneumonectomy. The authors hypothesized that an acute subclinical volume overload in these cases might be responsible for atrial fibrillation. Amar [35] found that patients who developed supraventricular tachycardia after lung resection had received, on average, 0.8 liters more fluid. This was significant on univariate but not on multivariate analysis.

3.8. Intraoperative hypotension and blood loss

Von Knorring [2] commented on the possible role of intraoperative hypotension, defined as a decrease in systolic blood pressure of 30% or more from the preoperative level, lasting at least 10 minutes. Thirty nine percent of patients who had intraoperative hypotension developed arrhythmias as opposed to 14% of those who did not have intraoperative hypotension (p <0.01). The occurrence of intraoperative hypotension may be related to surgical manipulation around the lung hilum and pericardium, which can cause intraoperative hypotension in 40-60% of patients studied [53]. Amar [35] reported that in a stepwise logistic regression analysis of correlates of post-operative supraventricular tachycardia in 100 patients undergoing pulmonary resection, an intraoperative blood loss of one liter or more was an independent risk factor with a relative risk of 3.5 (95% CI=1.2-10.5, p = 0.0001). On the other hand, Beck-Neilsen [21] did not find the magnitude of blood loss to be a predictor.

3.9. Anesthetic agents

Limited information is available as regards the risk of postoperative atrial fibrillation with specific anesthetic agents. On theoretical grounds, anesthetic agents have both proarrhythmic and anti-arrhythmic properties [54]. Halothane, enflurane and isoflurane depress sinus node automaticity; the resulting bradycardia may facilitate arrhythmias. These agents also increase atrial refractoriness, which may have an antiarrhythmic effect. Finally, halothane can promote reentry in ischemic ventricular fibers by increasing regional differences in action potential duration; it may be speculated that a similar effect occurs in atrial tissue. Mowry [14] found a higher incidence with cyclopropane (9%) or cyclopropane plus ether (11%) as compared to nitrous oxide (3%), but these are essentially descriptive data, as no statistical analysis was performed and no adjustment was made for the fact that patients given cyclopropane were older than those given nitrous oxide. Sorensen [53] found no difference between halothane and enflurane in a small study of 28 patients. Ritchie [31] also found no relation to anesthetic agent used. In any case, the half-life of anesthetic agents is short, and since most postoperative arrhythmias occur a few days after surgery, it is unlikely that the pharmacology of the anesthetic agent would play any substantial role in the genesis of postoperative atrial fibrillation.

4.0. Other factors

Epstein [9] reported that thyrotoxicosis was among the common associations of postoperative atrial fibrillation. Other factors assessed and not felt to be relevant in the development of postoperative atrial fibrillation include gender [5,18,32], antituberculous chemotherapy [14], medications given prior to surgery [5] , tobacco smoking [32] , indication for pneumonectomy [27], presenting symptoms [5], preoperative pulmonary function test results [2,25,32,35] , a history of angina [2], TNM surgical stage of cancer [27] , previous thoracic irradiation [27], need to complete chest wall resection [27], mediastinal shift from excessive fluid accumulation [9] , duration of operation [21] , the surgical technique of mass ligation at the hilum vs. individual ligation [5], occurrence of rapid mediastinal shift [5,7,23], hydrothorax [7], excess vagal nerve manipulation [5], anemia [5], transfusions [5] , febrile reactions [5] , serum potassium [21,23,31], or hypoxemia [23]. Von Knorring [2] also found no difference between the incidence from 1975 to 1982 vs 1983 to 1989, though patients with worse lung function underwent surgery in the latter period.

4. Mechanisms of Atrial Fibrillation after Noncardiac Thoracic Surgery

The etiologic factors responsible for the development of arrhythmias after thoracic surgery are uncertain. Several factors may play a role, either individually or in concert, including changes in vagal and sympathetic nervous activity, metabolic changes, atrial inflammation and the acute development of pulmonary hypertension and right heart dilatation.

4.1. Vagal effects

Atrial electrophysiologic properties are modulated by the autonomic nervous system. Changes in autonomic tone may influence the development of cardiac arrhythmias including atrial fibrillation [55] . For example, atrial fibrillation can be induced by the administration of acetylcholine or by vagal stimulation in a variety of mammalian experimental models [56-58]. Coumel [59] described a form of atrial fibrillation that occurs during conditions of heightened vagal tone. The mechanism by which vagal stimulation may facilitate atrial fibrillation is believed to be an inhomogenous decrease in atrial refractory period [60] which predisposes to reentrant wavelets.

Several authors have considered this a relevant mechanism. Bailey [4] suggested that vagal stimulation might be induced by infection of the bronchial stump or a stitch abscess following pneumonectomy; he speculated that this might then predispose to the development of atrial fibrillation. Sorensen [53] reported that 50% (14 of 28) of patients developed a fall in systolic blood pressure of 20 mmHg or more following traction on the pulmonary hilus; he attributed this to a vagal response. This is likely to occur in pulmonary surgery especially lung resection. Jakobsen [40] , on the other hand, in a study of the prophylaxis of arrhythmias after thoracotomy with metoprolol, reported that patients who later developed atrial fibrillation had in fact a trend to a higher heart rate throughout the postoperative period than those who did not develop atrial fibrillation; this suggested that vagal influence has a limited role to play in this post-operative setting.

4.2. Sympathetic stimulation

Sympathetic stimulation and catecholamine release may be expected to be triggered by the thoracotomy procedure or pain from the scar. Sympathetic excess may decrease the refractory period of the atria and increase ectopy; these effects may conceivably predispose to the development of atrial fibrillation. The argument for this is made most convincingly by Jakobsen [40]. In a study of the prophylactic effect of metoprolol on atrial fibrillation following lung resection, it was observed that patients who developed atrial fibrillation had a higher perioperative oxygen consumption (VO_2 122 mL/min/m^2 vs 74 mL/min/m^2, p<0.001) and postoperative cardiac index (4.0 ±1.0 L/min/m^2 vs. 3.4 ± 0.7 L/min/m^2 at 6 hr., p<0.01) than those who did not develop atrial fibrillation. In addition the heart rate was higher and the central venous pressure lower in patients who later developed atrial fibrillation. Prevention of atrial fibrillation with metoprolol further suggested that increased excitability caused by sympathetic activity may be a relevant etiologic factor.

4.3 Reduction in pulmonary vascular bed

Pneumonectomy leads to a reduction in the pulmonary vascular bed with possible subsequent elevation in the pulmonary pressure and acute development of cor pulmonale [8] . This may lead to atrial distension and/or changes in atrial pressure. In addition, loss of lung volume may lead to reduction in oxygenation and hypoxia.

A large number of studies have demonstrated a relation between the extent of lung resection and the incidence of postoperative atrial fibrillation (see above section). However, the high incidence of arrhythmias in thoracic surgery despite the absence of pulmonary tissue resection [3] suggests that though this mechanism probably explains the incremental risk with lung resection, the majority of cases of post-operative atrial fibrillation are due to other mechanisms.

4.4. Hypoxia

Following lung surgery, hypoxia related to loss of lung volume or underventilation may also make the atria more vulnerable to the development of atrial fibrillation. Hypoxia may also result in pulmonary vasoconstriction and therefore increase right ventricular systolic pressures; this could conceivably force the right ventricle to operate at a higher filling pressure and increase the right atrial pressures. Direct effects of hypoxia on atria may include a rise of atrial adenosine concentrations, which might shorten the atrial action potential, decrease the atrial refractory period and facilitate the induction of atrial fibrillation [61].

Attractive as this model may be, the clinical data suggests its role is modest. In a clinical report from the Mayo clinic [27] , arterial blood gases obtained just prior to or following the atrial dysrhythmias were reviewed; hypoxia (PaO_2 <60 mmHg) was observed in only 15% (8 of 53) and the arterial pH was not deranged in any. In a series of postoperative arrhythmias in 53 patients, Ritchie [31] could correlate the onset to hypoxia in only two. Similarly, on analysis of sixteen patients with postoperative atrial fibrillation, Ghosh [19] found arterial oxygen saturation <94% in only two patients. Adebo [23] reported that hypoxemia was not observed at the onset of arrhythmia following pneumonectomy. In Jakobsen's series[40], no patient who developed atrial fibrillation had an arterial oxygen saturation <94%; however, he suggested that the true contributing factor might be the oxygen supply/demand balance. In this report, all patients with an oxygen consumption higher than 100 mL/min/m^2 after induction of anesthesia and a postoperative oxygen consumption higher than 175 mL/min/m^2 developed atrial fibrillation.

4.5. Pericardial inflammation

Several series comment on autopsy evidence of pericarditis in patients who developed postoperative arrhythmias and subsequently died. Cerney [8] reported that of four patients who died, autopsy showed pericardial inflammation in two; this was localized to the atrium in one. Krosnick [6] found a small area of pericarditis in the one patient who died and had an autopsy. Epstein [9] found an extensive sero-fibrinous pericarditis in one of two patients who underwent autopsy after having had atrial fibrillation following pneumonectomy for lung cancer. In Massie's series [5] eleven patients had postoperative cardiac arrhythmias, three died and two were autopsied; both showed extensive pericarditis. Cohen [7] reported that autopsies were performed on six of fifteen patients who developed atrial arrhythmias post-thoracotomy; four showed metastatic tumor involving the epicardium and pericardium.

The animal sterile pericarditis model of atrial fibrillation is well described [49,50]. In a clinical study, Sorensen [53] reported that soft rubbing of the pericardium induced premature atrial complexes or a nodal rhythm in 15 of 28 patients studied. The incidence of atrial fibrillation is much higher following cardiac surgery, in which the pericardium is almost always entered, than in thoracic non-cardiac or non-thoracic surgery. Thus there is a sufficiently plausible biological hypothesis to suggest that this is a valid mechanism of postoperative atrial fibrillation. Its role in thoracic surgery, however, must be presumed to be small, given the evidence for lack of incremental effect of pericardial incision on the incidence of atrial fibrillation following pneumonectomy (see section above).

4.6. Atrial volume and pressure.

Right ventricular afterload may be increased in thoracic non-cardiac surgery by reduction of the pulmonary vascular bed and by hypoxia-induced pulmonary vasoconstriction. Both these mechanisms may secondarily result in higher right sided filling pressures. In addition, excessive administration of fluids may result in higher right atrial pressures. All these can result in atrial distention, which can alter the atrial electrophysiologic properties through stretch induced mechanisms [55]. Krumbhaar [62] noted an increased amplitude of the P wave following pulmonary artery ligature; this was presumably due to an acute increase in right heart pressures.

Consistent with this hypothesis, Lindgren [63] showed, in a hemodynamic study, that an increase in the central venous pressure and the right ventricular end-diastolic pressure on the first postoperative day was significantly ($p<0.05$) associated with the occurrence of atrial tachyarrhythmias on the second postoperative day. In addition, Krowka [27] found that atrial fibrillation occurred more frequently in patients who developed post-operative interstitial pulmonary edema. Amar [35] reported that in patients developing supraventricular tachycardia after pulmonary resection, postoperative echocardiography revealed a significant elevation of right ventricular pressure measured by the velocity of the tricuspid regurgitant jet when compared with patients without supraventricular tachycardia. Right atrial and ventricular dimensions and right atrial pressure were not different. A tricuspid regurgitant jet ≥ 2.7 m/s was associated with a relative risk of 3.6 (95%CI= 1.1-12.1, $p<0.05$) for postoperative supraventricular tachycardia in a multivariate analysis.

A dissenting voice is that of Jakobsen [40], who found that patients who later developed atrial fibrillation had a lower central venous pressure during the observation period. However, the difference, though statistically significant ($p<0.01$), was small in absolute terms (for example, 7 ± 3 mmHg vs 8 ± 5 mmHg at 6 hr. post surgery). In addition, patients who did not develop atrial fibrillation were primarily treated with metoprolol, which may increase filling pressures.

5. Time Course of Atrial Fibrillation After Surgery

Table 2 shows the observations of time of onset of postoperative atrial fibrillation made by several authors; the results are reasonably consistent. Sixty to eighty

TABLE 2

YEAR	AUTHOR	COMMENT
1943	Currens[3]	varied from d2-d18
1946	Massie[5]	55% on d3, all in w1
1955	Krosnick[6]	88% in w1
1957	Cerney[8]	most in w1, all in m1
1958	Epstein[9]	85% in w1
1961	Wheat[12]	60% by d3, 84% in w1
1964	Mowry[14]	60% by d3, 87% by d6
1968	Shields[16]	most on d3-4, all but one in w1
1973	Beck-Neilsen[21]	82% by d4
1979	Adebo[23]	mean 4d (range 1-21 d)
1987	Krowka[27]	95% by d6
1990	Ritchie[31]	most in first 24 h, half perioperative
1992	von Knorring[2]	47% on d2, 80% by d3
1993	Asamura[32]	41% on d2, 80% by d3
1995	Amar[35]	median d3 (range 0-10d)
1996	Terzi[38]	mainly on d2, 75% by d2
1997	Jakobsen[40]	average 2.9 days post-operative

d= day, w=week, m=month

percent of cases will occur by the fourth post-operative day and nearly all in the first week (Figure 2). A minor disagreement persists regarding intraoperative onset: Ritchie [31] found that half the cases occurred perioperatively, while others [2,5,32,36] reported that half their cases occurred on the second or third postoperative day. The identification of the time period with the highest incidence of arrhythmias is important in the assessment of the role of various predisposing factors, in the design of studies and in the identification of therapies to prevent the occurrence of arrhythmias. Burman [20] noted that postoperative arrhythmias occurred later in patients treated with digitalis, on postoperative day three to five, as opposed to those not treated with digitalis, in whom arrhythmias occurred on the day of surgery or the next day. Ritchie [31] reported that patients who underwent pneumonectomy were statistically more likely to develop arrhythmias in the first twenty-four hours after surgery than those who underwent other forms of lung surgery.

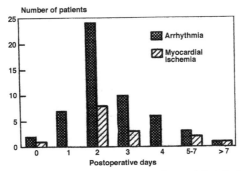

Figure 2. Distribution of postoperative cardiac events (arrhythmia and myocardial ischemia) in 53 patients by days after operation.
From Von Knorring et al, Ann Thorac Surg 1992; 53:642-7

6. Significance of Postoperative AF

6.1. Association with nonfatal events

Several authors have commented on the close association between postoperative arrhythmias and other complications. In Mowry's series [14], 7% of the patients developed a postoperative non-arrhythmic complication; of these 12% were associated with an arrhythmia as compared to 4% for the group as a whole. Cerney [8] commented that many of the patients with postoperative atrial fibrillation had empyema or pneumonia evident almost simultaneously. Associations described include mediastinal shift [14], collapse of the lung [3], change of posture [3], pericarditis [3], empyema [14], myocardial infarction [26] and repeat thoracotomy for bleeding [26]. Cardiac enzyme elevation and ECG changes were reported to precede dysrhythmias in 14% and follow dysrhythmias in another 14% of cases by Krowka [27]. In the same series, 45% of cases with dysrhythmia developed a ventricular rate in excess of 150 beats per minute and 38% dropped their systolic blood pressure by greater than 25% of baseline. It might be expected that series that confine the definition of atrial fibrillation to clinically relevant episodes would have a greater association with morbid events. On the other hand, Asamura [32] reported that only a third of patients with postoperative arrhythmias following thoracic surgery were symptomatic, while two-thirds were detected only on continuous ECG monitoring. Among 21 symptomatic patients, symptoms seen were palpitations (n=10), dyspnea (n=4), hypotension (n=3), chest discomfort (n=2), nausea (n=1) and disorientation (n=1).

6.2. Association with mortality

Some controversy exists regarding the relationship of postoperative atrial fibrillation to mortality. Krowka [27] reported that 25% of patients with dysrhythmia died compared to 7% of patients without dysrhythmia (p<0.001). Of sixteen postoperative deaths, 13 (81%) were associated with or preceded by dysrhythmias, and 69% (9/13) of these dysrhythmias were persistent or recurrent. Von Knorring [2] found that mortality rates were not different between those who remained in sinus rhythm and those who had single episodes of arrhythmia, however, those who developed persistent arrhythmia had a 17% mortality (3 of 18), as compared to a 2.4% mortality in pts without such arrhythmias (p<0.01). Shields [11] reported a series of 121 patients in whom 15 developed atrial fibrillation or flutter and 2 patients died with failure to control the arrhythmia, cardiac failure and concomitant respiratory insufficiency. Krosnick [6] and Epstein [9] each attributed two deaths to arrhythmia. Amar [35] reported a higher 30-day mortality in patients who developed supraventricular tachycardia after lung resection (17% versus 1%, p<0.02) as compared to patients who did not develop tachycardia. On the other hand, several authors [14,19,21,32,38] did not find any association of mortality and atrial arrhythmia. All the reports are essentially descriptive and only demonstrate an association of postoperative atrial fibrillation and mortality. Associated comorbid conditions are frequently present and the occurrence of arrhythmia may be an epiphenomenon; hence causality is unproven.

6.3. Relation to length of stay

Few authors have specifically looked at the role of atrial fibrillation in prolonging length of stay after thoracic noncardiac surgery. Wahi [30] reported a longer intensive care unit stay (4.8 days as compared to 2.5 days, p<0.05) and a longer hospital stay (13.7 days as compared to 9.3 days, p<0.05) in patients with postoperative atrial fibrillation as compared to those without postoperative arrhythmia. Amar [35] reported that patients who developed postoperative supraventricular tachycardia were more likely to be admitted to the intensive care unit (22% as compared to 1%, p<0.004) and had a longer hospital stay (22 days as compared to 10 days, p<0.02) as compared to those who did not develop tachycardia.

6.4. Recurrence and development of chronic AF

Most authors tend to agree that postoperative arrhythmias tend to be fleeting, often revert to sinus rhythm spontaneously and rarely develop into chronic arrhythmias. Currens [3] reported that 4 of 12 patients with postoperative atrial fibrillation or flutter had at least one further recurrence, but most spontaneously reestablished normal rhythm in 2-3 days. A similar 34% rate of persistence or recurrence was reported by von Knorring [2]. In Beck-Neilsen's report [21], 24% of patients with postoperative atrial fibrillation had a recurrent episode and all were in sinus rhythm on discharge from hospital. Asamura [32] reported that in only 5 of 63 cases (7%), the arrhythmia persisted for more than a week. Krowka [27] reported that 5% of patients with dysrhythmia were discharged in atrial fibrillation, and in Epstein's series [9], two patients went on to develop permanent atrial fibrillation; both had a prior history of paroxysmal atrial fibrillation. No patient in Cerney's study [8] went on to develop chronic atrial fibrillation.

7. Prevention of AF after Noncardiac Surgery

Table 3

DRUG	AUTHOR	YEAR	n	% AF W/DRUG	% AF W/O DRUG	P VALUE
Digitalis	Epstein[9]	1958	286	19	21	ns
	Wheat[12]	1961	439	12	23	0.01
	Bergh[15]	1967	229	9	20	<0.05
	Shields[16]	1968	125	3	14	n/a
	Juler[17]	1969	563	14	3	n/a
	Burman[20]	1972	207	4	14	n/a
	Adebo[23]	1979	68	12	45	n/a
	Ritchie[64]	1993	140	23	5	ns
Verapamil	Lindgren[63]	1991	25	0	31	<0.05
	Van Mieghem[36]	1996	199	8	15	ns
Metoprolol	Jakobsen[40]	1997	30	7	40	n/s
Magnesium	Terzi[38]	1996	200	11	27	0.008
Quinidine	Hurt[10]	1958	300	16	31	n/s
Flecainide	Borgeat[52]	1989	30	0	19	<0.01

ns=not significant, n/a=not available

Because of the high incidence of atrial arrhythmia and because of the potential associated morbidity and mortality, several investigators have attempted to use prophylactic antiarrhythmic therapy with mixed results. Table 3 lists relevant studies and results.

7.1. Digoxin

Several uncontrolled, nonrandomized, observational studies favor the role of digitalis in the prevention of atrial arrhythmias after thoracic noncardiac surgery. Shields and Ujiki [16] reported a nonrandomized study of 125 patients who underwent pulmonary surgery for malignancy; digitalis was administered prophylactically in 73. The incidence of postoperative atrial fibrillation was 14% in the control group and <3% in those receiving digitalis. Of note, continuous monitoring was not performed, and postoperative ECGs were recorded only every second day and as needed clinically; this may underestimate the true incidence as well as mask those with controlled ventricular rate. No toxicity was observed using a loading dose of 2-3 mg 2-3 days prior to surgery and 0.25 mg per day for 10-14 days. In another nonrandomized study, Burman [20] reported on 207 patients over 40 years old with normal hearts who underwent thoracotomy. Arrhythmias considered significant included atrial fibrillation, atrial tachycardia, atrial flutter, runs of premature ventricular beats, ventricular fibrillation and cardiac arrest. Arrhythmias occurred in 14% of control patients, and 4% of those on digitalis. Severe digitalis toxicity occurred in two patients. Arrythmias in the digitalis group were less frequent, less severe (easier to control) and occurred later. In an observational study [12] of digitalis in prevention of cardiac complications in 439 patients aged greater than 55 years who underwent major intra-thoracic surgery, Wheat and Buford reported a significantly lower rate (12% vs 23%, p=0.01) in the 137 pts who received digitalis. In a study of 68 pts undergoing pneumonectomy, Adebo [23] reported an incidence of arrhythmias (unspecified) of 45% in the 40 patients who did not receive digitalis as opposed to 21% in the 28 pts who did receive digitalis. Bergh [15] compared two nonrandomized groups of patients without heart disease who underwent pneumonectomy; postoperative atrial fibrillation occurred in 9% of patients treated with prophylactic digitalization and in 20% of those not treated.

On the other hand, several other uncontrolled, nonrandomized, observational studies reach the opposite conclusion. Juler [17] reported an observational study of 563 patients who underwent thoracic surgery from 1954-1966. The study was limited by the fact that patients who received digitalis averaged 10 years older than those who did not. The authors noted that the incidence of arrhythmias was fivefold higher and the incidence of mortality from cardiac arrhythmia was three-fold higher in patients who received digitalis, and felt it unlikely that the incidence could be explained away by the age difference. However, in the absence of statistical analysis to buttress this argument, the results must be interpreted with caution. The overall incidence of arrhythmia in the non-digitalized groups was low (<3%); in an uncontrolled study, it must be surmised that the high risk pts were given digoxin. Von Knorring [2] observed that preoperative therapy with digitalis or other antiarrhythmic drugs had been administered in 18% of those without arrhythmias and in 23% of those who did develop postoperative arrhythmia; the results were not statistically significant. In yet another uncontrolled study [9] 286 patients underwent surgery for lung cancer and the overall incidence of arrhythmia was 21%. Seventy patients received digitalis preoperatively; 19% of these developed an arrhythmia and the authors concluded that digitalis did not prevent disturbances of rhythm.

In 1990, Ritchie and colleagues [64] reported the results of a *randomized* trial of digoxin in 140 patients. Patients randomized to digitalis received two doses of 0.5 mg on the previous day, 0.25 mg with premedication and 0.25 mg per day for 9 days. The ECG was continuously monitored for four days. The incidence of atrial fibrillation was 23% in patients who received digitalis and 5% in those who did not; the difference was not statistically significant. In light of this data, it is now apparent that preoperative digitalization is not beneficial and may even be associated with its own complications [65]; thus prophylactic digitalization is no longer standard.

7.2. Verapamil

Limited data suggests that verapamil may have some role in the prevention of atrial fibrillation; the evidence is far from overwhelming. Lindgren [63] reported a study of 25 patients randomized in a double blind fashion, stratified by the extent of the operative procedure, to intravenous infusion of verapamil (0.01 mg/kg/hr followed by 80 mg tid PO) or placebo. Four of thirteen pts in the placebo group developed an atrial tachyarrhythmia (atrial fibrillation in 3 of 4). None in the verapamil group did so ($p<0.05$). Analysis of serial hemodynamic data showed that patients on verapamil had an attenuation of the hypoxic pulmonary vasoconstriction reflex and lower systolic right ventricular pressures; this may in part explain the mechanism of benefit. However, the control group was on average four years older; this was not adjusted for.

Van Meighem [36] reported that the incidence of atrial fibrillation in patients undergoing lobectomy or pneumonectomy was 8% in patients who received intravenous verapamil as opposed to 15 % in patients who received placebo (p=NS). The ventricular rate during atrial fibrillation in patients who received verapamil was 132 ± 22 bpm as opposed to 147 ± 22 bpm in those with placebo (p=NS). Verapamil was used in higher doses than in the above cited study, and had to be stopped in 25% of the patients due to bradycardia or hypotension. This result is not particularily convincing, but has a probability of a beta error, and so the findings may still be relevant [65]. A greater effect of verapamil might occur if side effects necessitating discontinuation were avoided. Nevertheless, the data do not support routine use of verapamil at this point.

7.3. Metopolol

In a small Danish study, Jakobsen and colleagues [40] randomized 40 patients to receive either metoprolol 100 mg before surgery and daily thereafter or placebo; 30

remained for analysis. Patients were typically followed by continuous electrocardiographic monitoring for 4 days and 3 daily ECGs for up to 10 days; episodes of atrial fibrillation lasting more than 30 seconds were included. Outside the continuous electrocardiographic monitoring period, diagnosis was based on 12 lead ECGs, often triggered by clinical symptoms. Atrial fibrillation developed in 7% of the metoprolol group and 40% of the placebo group ($p<0.05$). This is a small study, and enthusiasm for these results is tempered by the observation that atrial fibrillation was more often clinically recognized in the placebo group; this obviously may reflect effects on rate control rather than prevention of atrial fibrillation. Patients with lung disease may not tolerate beta blockade. Also, one patient who was receiving metoprolol developed pulmonary edema that required continued ventilation; this patient was excluded from analysis.

7.4. Magnesium

Terzi et al [38] reported on the use of infusion of magnesium sulfate on the prevention of tachyarrhythmias after thoracic noncardiac surgery. Two hundred patients were randomized; the treatment group received 2 grams of magnesium sulfate in 100 ml of 5% dextrose in water over 20 minutes at the thoracotomy and an additional 2 grams over 6 hours. The control group received either no treatment or, if aged over 70 or in cases of pneumonectomy or an intrapericardial procedure, digoxin (0.5 mg) starting on the day of surgery. Atrial tachyarrhythmias were seen in 11% of the treatment group and 27% of the control group ($p=0.008$). The majority of these arrhythmias were atrial fibrillation (90% in the treatment group and 85% in the control group). No true placebo group existed, and a deleterious effect of digoxin cannot be excluded from these results. The control group also had a slightly larger number of pneumonectomies and less wedge resections; at least part of the observed effect of magnesium may be attributed to this. Thus the data, though interesting, do not favor routine use of magnesium until further investigators confirm the validity of this approach.

7.5. Class I antiarrhythmic drugs

Other antiarrhythmic drugs have been used with anecdotal reports of success. In a case report in 1951, Philips [66] mentioned that the Massachusetts General Hospital Cardiovascular group had advocated the prophylactic use of quinidine preoperatively in all patients who were to undergo chest surgery. Many other surgeons at the time were in favor of using intravenous procaine or instilling procaine into the thoracic cavity in order to prevent reflex arrhythmia during the operation; he commented that these techniques were effective. In 1958, Hurt and Bates [10] reported the use of quinidine in 300 patients over the age of 45 years who underwent lung resection for malignancy. One hundred were randomized to oral quinidine or no drug, a placebo was not used. In this group, the incidence of atrial fibrillation and flutter in patients who received quinidine was 11% as compared to 31% in those who did not. Another 200 patients received quinidine in a non-randomized manner. The overall incidence of arrhythmia in patients who received quinidine was 16%. No patient developed a toxic reaction to quinidine. The authors concluded that quinidine was a valuable drug in the prevention of cardiac arrhythmia following lung resection. Limitations of this study are the absence of a placebo or blinding. In the absence of corroborative evidence from other studies, and given a potential pro-arrhythmic risk, we would not recommend routine use of quinidine in the preoperative setting.

The prophylactic value of flecainide (type 1C drug) in preventing arrhythmias after thoracic surgery was assessed in 30 patients by Borgeat et al [52]. Randomization was single-blind; 14 patients were given a loading dose of 2 mg/kg followed by 0.15 mg/kg/hr of intravenous flecainide and 16 patients received placebo. No atrial arrhythmias were observed on a 72 hour Holter recording in the flecainide treated group while 6 patients in the control group had to receive an antiarrhythmic drug (3 because of complex ventricular arrhythmia and 3 because of atrial fibrillation), $p<0.01$. However, this study should not be interpreted as demonstrating the effect of flecainide in reducing post operative atrial fibrillation; the statistical significance would not be maintained if only atrial fibrillation was considered. No side effects were noted.

7.6. Amiodarone

Van Mieghem [33] reported on the role of prophylactic amiodarone therapy after lung surgery in a prospective study, which was interrupted due to an unacceptably high incidence of adult respiratory distress syndrome in the amiodarone treated group. Amiodarone was administered as a bolus of 150 mg IV over 2 minutes, followed by 1200 mg per 24 hours for 3 days. Eleven (3 of 33) percent of patients treated with amiodarone developed adult respiratory distress syndrome; two died. No cases were observed in the remaining 64 patients who received either verapamil or placebo. On retrospective analysis of 552 patients at the same institution, the incidence of adult respiratory distress syndrome was 11% in the amiodarone group and <2% in the non-amiodarone group ($p<0.0001$).

The mechanism of adult respiratory distress syndrome is believed to be an interaction between amiodarone and high oxygen concentration in inspired air.

8. Nonthoracic Surgery

The segregation of noncardiac nonthoracic surgical procedures from other forms of surgery is appropriate for the following reasons. These procedures do not involve physical contact with the heart or associated structures thus eliminating the potential aggravating factors of inflammation, trauma, ischemia, etc. The procedures are a diverse group with a highly variable typical patient; include a multitude of surgical techniques; involve nonuniform postoperative management including monitoring and ECG recording, use of arrhythmogenic medications, and likelihood for aggravating coincidental factors; and have different durations of procedure and a variable duration and type of anesthesia.

The most comprehensive, and also contemporaneous, survey of all relevant aspects of postoperative supraventricular arrhythmias was undertaken by Polanczyk et al [1]. The results are important to review in detail and in juxtaposition to the little data available from the older literature. This consecutive series identified 4181 patients undergoing nonemergent noncardiac surgery at a single insititution; a new perioperative arrhythmia was detected in 317 patients (7.6%). The most common arrhythmia was AF, accounting for 54%. An undiagnosed SVT and atrial flutter were the next most common. The vast majority of arrhythmias were apparent by day 3 after surgery; only one third developed later during the hospitalization.

The clinical factors that were associated by multivariate analysis with supraventricular arrhythmia (AF analysis not performed separately) were older age, male gender, history of congestive heart failure or asthma, valvular disease on exam, previous history of supraventricular arrhythmia and premature atrial complexes on preoperative ECG, and American Society of Anesthesiologists class III or IV [1]. Intraoperative hypotension was also associated with an increased risk of AF. Many of these variables are risk factors for AF in the general population for AF after cardiac surgery.

Importantly, specific types of surgical procedures had a greater risk of arrhythmia: intrathoracic (discussed in detail in the sections above), abdominal aortic aneursym resection, other abdominal procedures and vascular procedures [1]. The highest risk was for the patient undergoing an intrathoracic procedure if not treated with digoxin, with an incidence of 24%, and a substantial increase in risk was also observed for those who had an abdominal aortic aneurysm resection, with an incidence of 16% . These associations were the result of a multivariate analysis and thus reflect factors that have an independent relationship to the designated endpoint.

Scattered other surgical series describe the frequency of postoperative AF. The results are variable and reflect the small sizes of the patient samples, general characteristics of surgical patient (i.e. risk factors), intensity of surveillance for arrhythmia, nonuniformity of endpoint description and other factors. The incidence varied from 5% in patients undergoing abdominal aortic surgery [67], 3% after joint arthroplasty [68], and well under 1% for resection of goiters [69], obesity surgery [70] and laparoscopy [71].

Like AF in other settings, clinical sequelae can include hemodynamic instability, congestive heart failure, myocardial ischemia, and a variety of other symptoms. Again as with AF in other settings, the most devastating consequence of AF is cerebrovascular accident [1,72]. AF also measurably increases the risk of myocardial infarction, ventricular tachycardia, cardiac arrest and other cardiac events [1]. These associations are not necessarily indicative of causation and it is quite possible that AF results from rather than precipitates many concurrent events. In this vein, AF was also associated with a higher risk of a variety of infections, pulmonary embolism and gastrointestinal bleeding [1].

The development of AF is associated with a prolongation of hospitalization, similar to observations after cardiac surgery. Polanczyk et al [1] calculated an addition of 2.5 days to length of stay, independent of other measured variables. This increment likely results from efforts to control the ventricular rate during AF, convert AF to sinus rhythm, treat complications and achieve therapeutic anticoagulation.

There is virtually no data on the prophylactic value of antiarrhythmic medications for AF after noncardiac nonthoracic surgery.

9. Conclusions

Atrial fibrillation is commonly seen after thoracic noncardiac surgery; the incidence from reported studies is, on average, 12-14%. Preoperative risk factors include age, lung malignancy, and preexisting cardiac disease. Operative risk factors include the extent of surgery, especially the volume of lung resected, and intraoperative hypotension. Postoperative risk factors include infections and volume overload. Mechanisms include changes in vagal and sympathetic nervous system activity, a reduction in the pulmonary vascular bed, hypoxia, pericardial inflammation and changes in atrial volume and pressure. Atrial fibrillation usually occurs in the first week, most often on the second or third postoperative day. Atrial fibrillation detected on continuous monitoring is usually asymptomatic. Symptomatic postoperative atrial fibrillation may be associated with comorbid events, especially lung infections and myocardial infarction, with an increased length of intensive care and hospital stay, and with mortality. Postoperative atrial fibrillation often reverts to sinus rhythm and rarely becomes chronic. Though there is some literature to support the use of digoxin, verapamil, metoprolol, magnesium and class I antiarrhythmic mediactions in prophylaxis, all the reported studies are either small, nonrandomised or uncorroborated by other investigators. Amiodarone appears to result in a high incidence of adult respiratory distress syndrome in this setting. Hence no prophylactic therapy can be unhesitatingly recommended.

Atrial fibrillation is also common after abdominal aortic aneurysm resection, other abdominal surgery and vascular procedures. Other surgical procedures have a much lower incidence of postoperative atrial fibrillation. Risk factors and clinical sequelae are similar to those for thoracic surgery. Studies on the prevention of atrial fibrillation in this setting are sorely needed.

References

1. Polanczyk CA, Goldmann L, Marcantonio ER, Orav EJ, Lee TH. Supraventricular arrhythmia in patients having noncardiac surgery: clinical correlates and effect on length of stay. Ann Intern Med 1998; 129: 279-285.
2. Knorring J, Lepantalo M, Lindgren L, Lindfors O. Cardiac arrhythmias and myocardial ishemia after thoracotomy for lung cancer. Ann Thorac Surg 1992;53:642-7.
3. Currens JH, White PD, Churchill ED. Cardiac arrhythmias following thoracic surgery. N Engl J Med 1943;229:360-4.
4. Bailey CC, Betts RH. Cardiac arrhythmias following pneumonectomy. N Engl J Med 1943;229:356-9.
5. Massie E, Valle AR, Cardiac arrhythmias complicating total pneumonectomy. Ann Intern Med 1947;26:231-9.
6. Krosnick A, Wasserman F. Cardiac arrhythmias in the older age group following thoracic surgery. Am J Med Sci 1955;230:541-50.

162

7. Cohen MG, Pastor BH. Delayed cardiac arrhythmias following non-cardiac thoracic surgery. Dis Chest 1957; 32:435.
8. Cerney CI. The prophylaxis of cardiac arrhythmias complicating pulmonary surgery. J Thorac Surg 1957;34:105-10.
9. Epstein EJ. Arrhythmias complicating the surgical treatment of lung carcinoma. British journal of Tuberculosis and Diseases of the Chest 1958; 52:195.
10. Hurt RL, Bates M. The value of quinidine in the prevention of cardiac arrhythmias after pulmonary resection. Thorax 1958; 13:39.
11. Shields TW. Factors influencing the morbidity and mortality in the older aged patient undergoing pulmonary surgery. Surg Gynec Obstet 1960; 111:598.
12. Wheat MW, Buford TH. Digitalis in surgery: extension of classical indications. J Thorac Cardiovasc Surg 1961; 41:162.
13. Catalayud JB, Kelser GA, Caseres CA. Incidence of cardiac arrhythmias following noncardiac surgery. J Thorac Cardiovasc Surg 1961; 41: 498.
14. Mowry FM, Reynolds EW Jr. Cardiac rhythm disturbances complicating resectional surgery of the lung. Ann Intern Med 1964;61:688-95.
15. Bergh NP, Dottori O, Malmberg R. Prphylactic digitalis in thoracic surgery. Scand J Resp Dis 1967; 48: 197.
16. Shields TN, Ujiki GT. Digitalisation for prevention of arrhythmias following pulmonary surgery. Surg Gynecol Obstet 1968.
17. Juler GL, Stemmer EA, Connolly SE. Complications of prophylactic digitalization in thoracic surgical patients. J Thorac Cardiovasc Surg 1969;58:t352-60.
18. Stougard J. Cardiac arrhythmias following pneumonectomy. Thorax 1969; 24:568.
19. Ghosh P, Pakrashi BC. Cardiac dysrhythmias after thoracotomy. Br Heart J 1972;34:474-6.
20. Burman SO. The prophylactic use of digitalis before thoracotomy. Ann Thorac Surg 1972;14:359-68.
21. Beck-Neilsen J, Rahbek Sorensen H, Alstrup P. Atrial fibrillation following thoracotomy for non-cardiac diseases, in particular cancer of the lung. Acta Med Scand 1973; 193:425-429.
22. Astrup P, Sorensen R. Metabolic studies following thoracotomy for lung cancer with particular reference to postoperative atrial fibrillation. Scand J Thorac Cardiovasc Surg 1975; 9:149-53.
23. Adebo OA, Singh AK. Digitalis in pneumonectomy and its implication. J Nat Med Assn 1979; 71:669.
24. Nagasaki F, Flehinger BJ, Martini N. Complications of surgery in treatment of carcinoma of the lung. Chest 1982;82:25-29.
25. Keagy BA, Schorlemmer GR, Murray GF, Starek PJK, Wilcox BR. Correlation of preoperative pulmonary function testing with clinical course inpatients after pneumonectomy. Ann Thorac Surg 1983;36:253-7.
26. Keagy BA. Pharr WF. Bowes DE. Wilcox BR. A review of morbidity and mortality in elderly patients undergoing pulmonary resection. Am Surg 1984; 50:213-6.
27. Krowka MJ, Pairolero PC, Trastek VF, Payne WS, Bernatz PE. Cardiac dysrhythmia following pneumonectomy: clinical correlates and prognostic significance. Chest 1987;91:490-5.
28. Mathisen DJ. Grillo HC. Wilkins EW Jr. Moncure AC. Hilgenberg AD. Transthoracic esophagectomy: a safe approach to carcinoma of the esophagus. Ann Thorac Surg 1988; 45:137-43.
29. Schwarz RE, Posner MC, Ferson PF, Keenan RJ, Landreneau RJ. Thoracoscopic techniques for the management of intrathoracic metastases. Results. Surg Endosc 1998; 12: 842-5.
30. Wahi R, McMurtney MJ, DeCaro LF et al. Determinants of perioperative morbidity and mortality after pneumonectomy. Ann Thor Surg 1989;48:33-7.
31. Ritchie AJ, Bowe P, Gibbons JRP. Prophylactic digitalization for thoracotomy: a reassessment. Ann Thorac Surg 1990;50:86.
32. Asamura H, Naruke T, Tsuchiya R, Goya T, Kondo H, Suemasu K. What are the risk factors for arrhythmias after thoracic operations. J Thorac Cardiovasc Surg 1993; 106:1104-1110.
33. Van Mieghem W, Coolen L, Malysse I, Lacquet L, Deneffe G, Demedts M. Amiodarone and the development of ARDS after lung surgery. Chest 1994;105:1642-45.
34. McDonald ML, Deschamps C, Ilstrup DM, Allen MS, Trastek VF, Pairolero PC. Pulmonary resection for metastatic breast cancer. Ann Thorac Surg 1994; 58:1599-602.
35. Amar D, Roistacher N, Burt M, Reinsel RA, Ginsberg RJ, Wilson RS. Clinical and echocardiographic correlates of symptomatic tachydysrhythmias after noncardiac thoracic surgery. Chest

1995; 108: 349-354.

36. Van Mieghem W, Tits G, Demuynck K, Lacquet L, Deneffe G, Tjandra-Maga T, Demedts M. Verapamil as prophylactic treatment for atrial fibrillation after lung operations. Ann Thorac Surg 1996; 61: 1083-6.

37. Allen MS, Deschamps C, Jones DM, Trastek VF, Pairolero PC. Video-assisted thoracic surgical procedures: the Mayo experience. *Mayo Clin Proc* 1996; 71:351-9.

38. Terzi A, Furlan G, Chiavacci P, Dal Corso B, Luzzani A, Dalla Volta S. Prevention of atrial tachyarrhythmias after non-cardiac thoracic surgery by infusion of magnesium sulfate. *Thorac Cardiovasc Surg* 1996; 44: 300-3.

39. Swanson SJ, Mentzer SJ, DeCamp MM Jr., Bueno R, Richards WG, Ingenito EP, Reilly JJ, Sugarbaker DJ. No-cut thoracoscopic lung plication: a new technique for lung volume reduction surgery. *J Am Coll Surg* 1997; 185:25-32.

40. Jacobsen CJ, Bille S, Ahlburg P, Rybrol L, Hjortholm R, Andresen EB. Perioperative metoprolol reduces the frequency of atrial fibrillation after thoracotomy for lung resection. J Cardiothorac Vasc Anesth 1997;11:746-51.

41. Benjamin EJ, Levy D, Vaziri S, D'Agostino RB, Belanger AJ, Wolf PA. Independent risk factors for atrial fibrillation in a population-based cohort. The Framingham Heart Study. J Am Med Assoc 1994; 271:840-4.

42. Leitch JW, Thomson D, Baird DK, Harris PJ. The importance of age as a predictor of atrial fibrillation and flutter after coronary artery bypass grafting. J Thorac Cardiovasc Surg 1990;100:338-42.

43. Mathew JP, Parks R, Savino JS, Friedman AS, Koch C, Mangano DT, Browner WS. Atrial fibrillation following coronary artery bypass graft surgery: predictors, outcomes, and resource utilization. Multicenter Study of Perioperative Ischemia Research Group. J Am Med Assoc 1996 ;276:300-6.

44. Almassi GH, Schowalter T, Nicolosi AC, Aggarwal A, Moritz TE, Henderson WG, Tarazi R, Shroyer AL, Sethi GK, Grover FL, Hammermeister KE. Atrial fibrillation after cardiac surgery: a major morbid event?. Ann Surg 1997;226:501-513.

45. Aranki SF, Shaw DP, Adams DH, Rizzo RJ, Couper GS, VanderVliet M, Collins JJ Jr, Cohn LH, Burstin HR. Predictors of atrial fibrillation after coronary artery surgery. Current trends and impact on hospital resources. Circulation 1996;94:390-7.

46. Gerson MC, Hurst JM, Hertzberg VS, Baugham R, Rouan GW, Ellis K. Prediction of cardiac and pulmonary complications related to elective abdominal and noncardiac thoracic surgery in geriatric patients. Am J Med 1990;88:101-7.

47. Breyer RH. Zippe C. Pharr WF. Jensik RJ. Kittle CF. Faber LP. Thoracotomy in patients over age seventy years: ten-year experience. J Thorac Cardiovasc Surg 1981; 81:187-93.

48. Szentmiklosi AJ, Nementh M, Szegi J, Papp JG, Szekeres L. On the possible role of adenosine in the hypoxia-induced alteration sof the electrical and mechanical activity of the atrial myocardium. *Arch Int Pharmacodyn* 1979; 238: 283-95.

49. Page P, Plumb VJ, Okumura K, Waldo AL. A new model of atrial flutter. J Am Coll Cardiol 1986; 8:872-879.

50. Kumagai K, Khrestian C, Waldo AL. Simultaneous multisite mapping studies during induced atrial fibrillation in the sterile pericarditis model. Insights into the mechanism of its maintainance. Circulation 1997; 95:511-21.

51. Craig SR, Walker WS. Initial experience of video assisted thoracoscopic pneumonectomy. *Thorax* 1995; 50: 392-5.

52. Borgeat A, Biollaz J, Bayer-Berger M, Kappenberger L, Chapuis G, Chiolero R. Prevention of arrhythmias by flecainide after noncardiac thoracic surgery. Ann Thorac Surg 1989;48:232-34.

53. Sorensen O, Waaben KB, Skovsted P. The incidence of cardiac arrhythmias and arterial hypotension subsequent to standardized surgical stimuli in patients undergoing thoracotomy with special reference to enflurane and halothane. Acta Anaesthesiol Scand 1986;30:630-2.

54. Atlee JL, Bosnjak ZJ. Mechanisms for cardiac dysrhythmias during anesthesia. Anesthesiology 1990;72:347.

55. Waxman MB, Wald RW, Cameron D. Interaction between the autonomic nervous system and tachycardias in Main Cardiology Clinics 1983 Vol 1, No2 p 143-184.

56. Burn JH, Vaughan-Williams EM, Walker JM. Effects of acetyl-choline in heart lung preparation including production of auricular fibrillation. J Physiol (London) 1953;128:277-293.

57. Loomis TA, Krop S. Auricular fibrillation induced and maintained by acetylcholine or vagal stimulation. Circ Res 1955;3:390-396.

58. Higgnis CB, Vatner SF, Braunwald E. Parasympathetic control of the heart. Pharmacol Rev

164

1973;25:119-155.

59. Coumel P, Attuel P, Lavallee Flammang D. Syndrome d'arrhythmie aruriculaire d'origine vagal. Arch Mal Coeur 1978;71:645-658.

60. Alessi R, Nusynowitz M, Abdilskov JA. Non-uniform distribution of vagal effects on the atrial refractory period. Am J Physiol 1958;194:406-410.

61. Bertolet BD, Hill JA, Kerensky RA, Belardinelli L. Myocardial infarction related atrial fibrillation: role of endogenous adenosine. Heart 1997; 78: 88-90.

62. Krumbhaar EB. Note on electrocardiographic changes following acutely increase pressure following pulmonary artery ligature. AM J Med Sci 1934, Vol clxxxvi (127) 792-794 quoted in Massie [5].

63.Lindgren L, Lepantalo M, Von Knorring J, Rosenberg P, Orko R, Scheinin B. Effect of verapamil on right ventricular pressure and atrial tachyarrhythmia after thoracotomy. Br J Anaesth 1991;66:205-11.

64. Ritchie AJ, Tolan M, Whiteside M, et al. Prophylactic digitalization fails to control dysrhythmia in thoracic surgical operations. Ann Thorac Surg 1993; 55:86-88.

65. Little AG. invited comment on Van Mieghem W et al. Verapamil as prophylactic treatment for atrial fibrillation after lung operations. Ann Thorac Surg 1996; 61: 1086.

66. Phillips E. Delayed Cardiac arrhythmias following pneumonectomy. Ann West Med & Surg 1951; 778-781.

67. von Knorring J, Lepantalo M, Hietanen H, Peder M. Predicting of postoperative cardiac events using ambulatory ECG monitoring prior to abdominal aortic surgery. Eur J Vasc Endovasc Surg 1995; 9:133-7.

68. Kahn RL. Hargett MJ. Urquhart B. Sharrock NE. Peterson MG. Supraventricular tachyarrhythmias during total joint arthroplasty. Incidence and risk. Clin Orthop 1993; (296):265-9.

69. Allo MD. Thompson NW. Rationale for the operative management of substernal goiters. Surgery 1983; 94:969-77.

70. Ramsey-Stewart G. The perioperative management of morbidly obese patients (a surgeon's perspective). Anaesth Intensive Care 1985; 13:399-406.

71. Sand J, Marmela K, Airo I, Nordback I. Staging of abdominal cancer by local anesthesia outpatient laparoscopy. Hepato-Gastroenterology 1996;43(12):1685-8.

72. Parikh S. Cohen JR. Perioperative stroke after general surgical procedures. N Y State J Med 1993; 93:162-5.

INDEX